"Manny is a voice that our generatio[...]

Zach Windahl, author, *The Bible Study*

"Manny Arango is not just an outstanding communicator, he is an exceptional human being. I have watched him walk through tragedy and loss with the same spiritual resilience that keeps him anchored in his success. *Brain Washed* is more than a great book; it is a conversation with a great young leader on how to frame your future."

Dr. Terry Crist, lead pastor, City of Grace, Phoenix/Tucson/Las Vegas

"Reading this book helped me realize how important the message that Manny is presenting is for the generation we live in. Sometimes we all allow trauma and pain to determine how we journey through life and relationships. *Brain Washed* is a clear guide to get the right perspective. This book is necessary, and the step-by-step guides for overcoming trauma and taking thoughts captive will help us take control of our minds."

Chandler Moore, worship leader, Maverick City Music

"Manny is a much-needed voice in the church today, and *Brain Washed* is an excellent addition to Manny's growing library of resources. Get *Brain Washed*!"

Nathan Finochio, founder, TheosU

"Manny is not only a gifted preacher and communicator, but a needed thinker and brilliant mind in the body of Christ. This book is not simply theological theory, but is born out of Manny's renewed mind and love for God's Word. *Brain Washed* will be a gift to a new generation of believers who are ready to take their thinking to the next level!"

Pastor Jabin Chavez, City Light Church, Las Vegas

"Manny Arango is the epitome of the song 'Enemy's Camp.' He will crawl through hell to get it back. This book is just a synopsis of the life he has led for many years. It's an honor to call him a friend and an inspiration. Share this after you read it."

Tim Somers, central youth pastor, Elevation Church

"Manny Arango is an educated, modern-day theologian with the pastoral, missionary, and evangelistic experience to be the exact kind of teacher and thinker to capture the true challenge of using Scripture to rightly divide soul and spirit, joint and marrow. This book is a MUST for the modern-day believer!"

Pastor Andy Thompson, senior pastor and founder, World Overcomers Christian Church

"Manny Arango is a rising voice for today's generation. He is a bold, biblical, insightful preacher and now a writer. *Brain Washed* deals with relevant issues from a scriptural standpoint. A book for all mankind!"

Frank Damazio, author, *The Making of a Leader*

"Manny Arango has written a timely and relevant book to help the body of Christ find lasting freedom from toxic thought patterns. Manny has managed to integrate deep biblical and theological truth with relatable storytelling in a writing style that is profound and enjoyable. *Brain Washed* is a necessary message and a must-read book for every believer."

Pastor Robert Madu, Social Dallas

"I'm so excited for people to read *Brain Washed*. This message of mind renewal and mental freedom is so needed and will set so many people free from the prison of negative thoughts they've been trapped in. I honestly believe that Manny Arango is a voice to our generation and his perspective on mental health is wise, practical and godly."

Pastor Taylor Madu, Social Dallas

BRAIN WASHED

BRAIN WASHED

Overcome Toxic Thoughts and Take Back Control of Your Mind

MANNY ARANGO

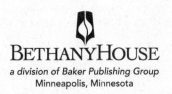

BETHANYHOUSE

a division of Baker Publishing Group
Minneapolis, Minnesota

© 2022 by Emmanuel Arango

Published by Bethany House Publishers
11400 Hampshire Avenue South
Minneapolis, Minnesota 55438
www.bethanyhouse.com

Bethany House Publishers is a division of
Baker Publishing Group, Grand Rapids, Michigan

Printed in the United States of America

Library of Congress Cataloging-in-Publication Data
Names: Arango, Manny, author.
Title: Brain washed : overcome toxic thoughts and take back control of your
    mind / Manny Arango.
Description: Minneapolis, Minnesota : Bethany House, a division of Baker
    Publishing Group, 2022.
Identifiers: LCCN 2022013948 | ISBN 9780764240690 (paperback) | ISBN
    9780764241215 (casebound) | ISBN 9781493437894 (ebook)
Subjects: LCSH: Thought and thinking—Religious aspects—Christianity.
Classification: LCC BV4598.4 .A73 2022 | DDC 153.4/2—dc23/eng/20220414
LC record available at https://lccn.loc.gov/2022013948

Unless otherwise indicated, Scripture quotations are from THE HOLY BIBLE,
NEW INTERNATIONAL VERSION®, NIV® Copyright © 1973, 1978, 1984, 2011 by
Biblica, Inc.® Used by permission. All rights reserved worldwide.

Scripture quotations identified NKJV are from the New King James Version®.
Copyright © 1982 by Thomas Nelson. Used by permission. All rights reserved.

This book recounts events in the life of Emmanuel Arango according to the
author's recollection and from the author's perspective. While all the stories
are true, some dialogue and identifying details have been changed to protect
the privacy of the people involved.

Cover design by LOOK Design Studio

Emmanuel Arango is represented by the literary agency A Drop of Ink, LLC,
www.adropofink.pub.

Baker Publishing Group publications use paper produced from sustainable for-
estry practices and post-consumer waste whenever possible.

23 24 25 26 27 28   7 6 5 4 3 2

To my wife, Tia

The journey required of us to become parents, forced us to practice the principles found in this book. Each year we waited to become parents I witnessed your adopting the Mind of Christ. Thank you for being mentally strong and choosing faith.

To my son, Theophilus

I wrote every chapter of this book knowing you'd read them one day. Even when doctors told us conceiving was impossible, I still wrote.

Contents

Introduction

THE FINGER OF GOD

For although they knew God, they neither glorified him as God nor gave thanks to him, but their thinking became futile and their foolish hearts were darkened. Although they claimed to be wise, they became fools.

Romans 1:21–22

I WAS IN A TRANCE as I stared at the ceiling of the Sistine Chapel. Countless photographs of Michelangelo's famous fresco *Creation of Adam* exist, yet as I stood under the majestic work of art, I realized I had never truly seen the mural before that moment. No photograph can fully capture Michelangelo's three-dimensional effects. The images pop and pulsate with character, and the longer I stared, the more it felt as though Adam and God were moving closer and closer toward the crowd gathered beneath them.

It took my breath away.

Our tour guide startled me, and I immediately regretted that after standing in line for hours in peak-summer heat to enter the

Vatican City State, I had bolted off on my own, face like flint, leaving my group behind. But now that he'd found me, the guide pointed out that the shape of the swooping scarlet robe behind God forms an outline of the human brain and a green portion of fabric outlines the shape of the brain stem. He also drew my attention to how Adam's expression, depicted prior to his receiving God's touch, doesn't simply lack life but intelligence as well.

I was in awe of Michelangelo's ability to convey a rich theological message through art. When God created humanity, He endowed it with His divine image by granting us the gift of rational thought, intellectual creativity, and consciousness. To Michelangelo, then, it seems the divine spark that separated humans from other creatures in the garden of Eden was the power of their minds. God desires relationship and intimacy with humanity, and therefore He created Adam as a rational and intelligent being, one who could receive and reciprocate love and understanding.

The brilliance of Adam's mind is immediately on display as he goes to work studying God's creation within the opening chapters of Genesis. The Bible tells us that Adam is given the task of naming and categorizing all the species of animal life found in the garden of Eden. Earth is colonized and ruled by heaven through the image-bearing brilliance of Adam.

Did you know everyone's brains are washed—either by the Serpent or by God, our Father and King? But whereas the Serpent wants to destroy us with his brain washing, God wants to wash our brains with His truth. And we allow Him to do that by abandoning the Mind of Adam and adopting the Mind of Christ.

In the same way a criminal is incentivized to kidnap the son or daughter of wealthy parents, the Serpent's assault on Adam and Eve was a direct attack against God Himself. He kidnapped and hijacked Adam and Eve's minds in order to throw the entire colony of Earth into rebellion, and we are all part of that war. The Serpent's goal is to destroy God's kingdom, so he continues his assault on God's throne by releasing a virus into the Mind of Adam.

This book is a field guide to help you win the battle taking place in the trenches of your mind, to regain control over rogue thoughts, so the kingdom of heaven can be firmly established on Earth. The dominion you experience over your mind directly correlates to the dominion heaven has on this planet. Your thought life will either be host to the terrorist cells of the Serpent or claimed as an instrument of righteousness that God can mobilize for His purposes. You will either be brain washed by the Serpent's secular agenda or brain washed in the blood of the Lamb. There is no neutral territory.

You may currently view your mind as your private property. You may believe that the thoughts you entertain have no effect on others. You may have picked up this book for self-help or self-improvement. But the truth of the matter is that our minds are valuable real estate, and the King is constantly giving us opportunities to surrender them to Him so they can be available for His use. The Serpent, though, desperately wants to privatize your mind, and the over-individualization of our culture is part of his scheme to push our species toward independence, insecurity, and isolation. That's why we must unconditionally surrender our minds to God instead of using them to oppose His rule.

The Never-Ending Fall

The realness of Michelangelo's *Creation of Adam* matches the painful images of the fall of Adam and Eve. Adam and his bride were deceived by the Serpent and ate from the Tree of Knowledge of Good and Evil. The Bible describes what follows as the fall of humankind.

Canyons were hollowed out as these first people fell to the ground. The flat earth beneath them cracked as the weight of glory crashed and crumbled. God's mirrored image imploded and shattered within them like a thousand glass windows on the surface of a skyscraper. The sound of Adam's knee hitting the garden floor echoed throughout creation like thunder. Their physical fall, however, was only a reflection of their mental collapse.

Their brilliance was darkened.

Their intelligence was muted.

Their understanding faded.

Their genius disintegrated.

The apostle Paul taught the Roman church that when humanity refuses to acknowledge God as the Creator and King, our thinking is directly affected by that choice. Like a lamp that isn't connected to a source of electricity, our minds are dark without the light of God. The same pattern we find with Adam and Eve is clearly at work with all people. Paul wrote, "Although they knew God, they neither glorified him as God nor gave thanks to him, but their thinking became futile and their foolish hearts were darkened. Although they claimed to be wise, they became fools" (Romans 1:21–22). In a quest to gain worldly understanding, these humans ended up destroying the very minds they sought to enhance.

Unfortunately, many of us have embarked on this same journey of self-improvement. Many of us are also still operating with the fallen and debased Mind of Adam. Every mental stronghold you may have experienced in your lifetime is the result of Adam and Eve's fall from glory. We can live in the caverns and dark caves carved out by their fall, or we can ascend the mountain of the Lord to adopt His thoughts and His mind.

This book is for all the hitchhikers trying to leave the deserted minds of Adam and Eve behind.

iOS—The Mind of Christ

Years ago, I visited an Apple Store because my laptop was running really slow. Some friends had told me about a new operating system, and I asked the "Apple Genius" if he could upgrade my software. He checked out my computer and then broke the unfortunate news that the upgraded software wasn't compatible with my older laptop. To get a new operating system, I would have to part ways with my old laptop and get a new one. In other words, new software required new hardware.

I'm afraid a lot of Christian teaching surrounding the life of the mind encourages people to upgrade their software while still using Adam's hardware. But the Mind of Christ is the new model, and God's operating system is compatible only with a complete change of hardware.

Jesus echoed this idea when He said, "Neither do people pour new wine into old wineskins. If they do, the skins will burst; the wine will run out and the wineskins will be ruined. No, they pour new wine into new wineskins, and both are preserved" (Matthew 9:17). I have often made the mistake of trying to put God's thoughts into the Mind of Adam, and although there is an improvement, it's only temporary. Jesus doesn't simply want to give us new thoughts; He secured and promises us a new mind. Through the work of the Holy Spirit in our lives, Jesus can always deliver new thoughts to our human minds. His thoughts, however, are most compatible with His mind—the Mind of Christ.

Might I add that I took my Apple product to an Apple Store because the manufacturer was authorized, equipped, and the most knowledgeable concerning the product. As I looked up at the ceiling of the Sistine Chapel, I was reminded of a simple truth—God is the manufacturer of the human mind and consciousness, yet humanity isn't always convinced that He's the best equipped or the most knowledgeable source for how to heal the mind.

In this book we will hold open the Bible as an instruction manual for the human mind and learn what this ancient God has to say about our current dilemmas. God's Word, and in particular the New Testament, isn't provided merely as an attempt to improve your mind but rather as an invitation for you to adopt the Mind of

Christ. The old hardware has reached its limit for upgrades. The old wineskins have been stretched to capacity. We've tried to make our own minds stronger, but honestly, we were all born with the Mind of Adam, our fallen forefather. We didn't do anything wrong; we made no mistakes. We were simply born into the lineage of Adam and inherited a flawed mind because of his decision to accept the Serpent's thought.

That's not where the story ends, though. The good news is that there's a bridge between the Mind of Adam, which we are all born into, and the Mind of Christ, which we all have access to. The Bible outlines a road map across that bridge, moving from that old mind to the new. From that fallen mind to the exalted one. From that natural mind to the supernatural.

Worth It but Not Easy

It's not easy leaving the familiarity of Adam's mind where we are all well-learned scholars and experts. Nor is navigating the Mind of Christ easy, because it is indeed foreign terrain. But I believe we can get there—especially if we journey together.

Nor is the renewal of our minds instant or quick but rather a life-long process. Moving from the depraved Mind of Adam to adopting the glorious and brain washed Mind of Christ is, as I've also indicated, a journey. But again, the good news is that Scripture lays out a road map for us to follow, which means we can track our progress along the way.

I desperately wish I could provide a shortcut to help us all arrive at the Mind of Christ quickly. But what I can do is offer a process and a companion along the narrow path to the Mind of Christ.

I also wish we could immediately skip ahead to the sections of this journey that are more practical. But to unravel the complex cords of consciousness that have led us to our current mindsets, we must retrace the steps of our fallen foreparents. The opening chapters of Genesis outline the tragic fall of Adam and Eve, but in their fall, they left behind bread crumbs that will help us restore our minds to their original factory settings. The Gospels also outline this pattern since Christ is indeed a second Adam, sent to live out the course of the first Adam's life as an archetype for the rest of humanity. On this journey, we will backtrack in order to retrace the fallen steps of Adam, and then we'll move forward to follow the steps of Jesus.

The fall of Adam and Eve was layered, thus the foundation for the Mind of Christ is layered. Adam and Eve sustained three layers of destruction, and we'll have to construct three layers of foundation in order to recover all that was lost.

The first layer to sustain significant damage was their concept of God. Second, the Serpent destroyed their understanding of self. Last, their ability to relate to each other was marked with distrust, doubt, and dysfunction. And as we retrace the fall of humanity, we'll see these three distinct thought patterns. The Serpent's deception begins with a toxic thought about God. The fruit immediately shatters their understanding of self. And last, the Serpent positions humans against one another.

All toxic thoughts can be organized into those three categories:

1. Thoughts about God
2. Thoughts about self
3. Thoughts about others

The first stops along the journey may not seem as immediately helpful as the latter stops, but as your tour guide, I promise that the foundation we establish in the following chapters will support the weight of everything we endeavor to build. When we stand inside a home or building, we rarely compliment the owners or architects on how impressive we find the foundation. The foundation is of utmost importance but goes unnoticed, taken for granted, and unpraised.

If we are to stand on the balcony of a renewed mind, hang expensive curtains from the windows of changed perspective, or enjoy the peaceful gardens of healed memories, then we must first pour the concrete for a stable and permanent foundation. We may never compliment builders on how perfectly level we find their foundations, but we sure would notice and complain if the foundations were faulty. For all you *Fixer Upper* fans, TV's Chip Gaines must do some structural demolition before Joanna Gaines can order furniture and fill the home with aesthetics and decor.

A Mind Map

I have carefully mapped out our journey from the Mind of Adam to the Mind of Christ.

Independence → Intimacy

Insecurity → Identity

Isolation → Interdependence

Independence from God → Intimacy with God

Insecurity within self → Identity within self

Isolation from others → Interdependence with others

The Mind of Adam is marked by independence, insecurity, and isolation, and so chapters 1, 2, 3, and 4 explain those mental frameworks. In order to build upward, we must first secure some bulldozers and dig down into the fallen Mind of Adam.

The Mind of Christ moves us from independence to intimacy, from insecurity to identity, and from isolation to interdependence. Chapters 5 and 6, then, outline the Mind of Christ—the human archetype for intimacy, identity, and interdependence. This is where we'll construct the pillars, beams, walls, HVAC, and plumbing of our structure.

The last part of this book—chapters 7, 8, and 9—explores more practical thought patterns, like memories, regret, and anxiety. This final section is where we will furnish our home and install a security system for lasting protection.

Let's begin.

PART ONE

Understanding the Mind of Adam

1

Doubt Takes the Lead

What comes into our minds when we think about God is the most important thing about us.[1]

A.W. Tozer

When [Satan] undertook to draw Eve away from God, he did not hit her with a stick, but with an idea.[2]

Dallas Willard

I FELT LIKE A COMPLETE FAILURE as one of my students stood suffering from a crippling panic attack in the lobby of our church minutes before the worship service was to begin. A massive boa constrictor of anxiety had coiled itself around her, and prayer seemed useless as I watched her struggle to breathe. She was bent over, trapped under the pressure, and I felt powerless to protect her from this generational Goliath.

Over the previous decade, as hundreds and thousands of young people poured into our church, we quickly learned that many of them were terrorized by mental health challenges and plagued with destructive thought patterns. Statistically, we who lead and minister to these young people are doing so to the most medicated generation in the history of America.

I've prayed with teenagers who were drowning in depression.

I've talked with suicidal middle schoolers.

I've counseled young adults who constantly compared themselves to others.

I've sat with entire families trapped in a maze of toxic thoughts.

And I've stood in the lobby as a student got hit with a panic attack. (After a couple of minutes, my wife, who suffered from anxiety attacks for years, came to the rescue and helped restore this young girl's peace of mind.)

There's tension between the real and raw experiences I've had with people and the Bible I'm typically holding in my hand during those experiences. God's Word is clear regarding the realm of the mind and the power of our thoughts. The entire canon of Scripture is filled with promises and lessons on mental freedom, clarity, and peace.

Second Timothy 1:7 declares, "God has not given us a spirit of fear, but of power and of love and of *a sound mind*" (emphasis mine, NKJV).

Second Corinthians 10:5 teaches, "We demolish arguments and every pretension that sets itself up against the knowledge of God, and *we take captive every thought* to make it obedient to Christ" (emphasis mine).

Philippians 4:6 says, "Do not be *anxious* about anything, but in every situation, by prayer and petition, with thanksgiving, present your requests to God" (emphasis mine).

In just these three short verses, the Bible teaches us that God has given us the power of sound thinking, the ability to take every thought captive, and dominion over anxiety and anxious thoughts. The gospel of Jesus Christ includes the cleansing of our minds, the renewal of our thoughts, and the power to operate the complex machinery of our minds with expertise and care. When we accept Christ as our Lord and Savior, He washes our minds in His blood and gives us a new mind.

In other words, He brain washes us.

The prophet Isaiah assures us that Jesus was "pierced for our transgressions," "crushed for our iniquities," and that "by his wounds we are healed" (Isaiah 53:5). We have access to the healing grace of God because Jesus was wounded in our place. This verse is the epitome of good news, but the good news gets even better when we examine the wounds of Christ and the corresponding areas of healing where we can exercise faith.

By His wounds, we are healed.

- Jesus was circumcised so we could be healed of private pain.
- Jesus's sweat turned to blood to heal the human will.
- Jesus was whipped across His back so our past can be healed.
- Jesus was pierced in His side so our relationships can be healed.
- Jesus's feet were wounded to restore the authority that was Adam's.
- Jesus's hands were nailed so our hands may receive our inheritance.
- Lastly, Jesus wore a crown of thorns so our minds may be healed.

The first bread crumb our foreparents left for our journey was their unfortunate conversation with the Serpent, so let's start there.

Hit with an Idea

Genesis 3:1–5 says,

Now the serpent was more crafty than any of the wild animals the LORD God had made. He said to the woman, "Did God really say, 'You must not eat from any tree in the garden'?" The woman said to the serpent, "We may eat fruit from the trees in the garden, but God did say, 'You must not eat fruit from the tree that is in the middle of the garden, and you must not touch it, or you will die.'" "You will not certainly die," the serpent said to the woman. "For God knows that when you eat from it your eyes will be opened, and you will be like God, knowing good and evil."

The late Dallas Willard, who had a brilliant theological mind, offered eye-opening commentary on how the Serpent was able to seduce Eve. In his classic book *Renovation of the Heart*, he wrote,

> Ideas and images are, accordingly, the primary focus of Satan's efforts to defeat God's purposes with and for humankind. When we are subject to his chosen ideas and images, he can take a nap or a holiday. Thus, when he undertook to draw Eve away from God, he did not hit her with a stick but with an idea. It was with the idea that God could not be trusted and that she must act on her own to secure her own well-being.[3]

The Serpent understood that ideas and thoughts were weapons that could be used for the destruction of God's kingdom and creation. The first thought he held out for Adam and Eve as bait was doubt. He knew if they doubted the character of God, they would be compelled to become self-sufficient beings, so he convinced them that their King was a dictator, making the fight for independence inevitable. He knew if those first humans chose independence, God would not allow them to secede from the union without a war. (The Serpent also knew peace wouldn't be available for my anxious teenager in the lobby of our church because of the war-torn creation.) The first domino fell as Eve reached out her hand, and the human race is still tripping over and being crushed under the dominoes as they continue to fall.

The Serpent didn't destroy Adam and Eve with fruit; their undoing was a rather cruel and simple thought. And until we address that thought, our minds will be filled with countless other toxic thoughts. The first foundational stone of the Mind of Adam is doubt, specifically doubt in the character of God. The Mind of Adam does not trust God; it's at war with Him. And unfortunately, although countless numbers of people today eagerly desire the peace of God, their minds are at war with God too. That makes it impossible for them to *have* the peace of God because they must first *be* at peace with God.

The root of anxiety is deeply spiritual. My student in the lobby, hyperventilating and filled with angst, represents the fallout of our war with God, and until there's unconditional surrender, there will be a continual onslaught of anxiety in our broken world.

Unconditional surrender, however, is possible only when we trust in the character and goodness of our Creator and King. The Serpent works tirelessly to continue casting the shadow of doubt and distrust on humanity's perception of God, and as we walk in the footsteps of our fallen foreparents, our minds are filled with more and more doubt.

Conversely, the first foundational stone of the Mind of Christ is faith, belief, and trust. As we determine to make our first move from the Mind of Adam to the Mind of Christ, we must move from doubt and independence to trust and surrender.

Doubting God's True Character Is Heretical

The Serpent stands before Eve and poses a question designed to produce doubt and mistrust: "Did God really say, 'You must not eat from any tree in the garden'?" (Genesis 3:1).

The cunning and crafty Serpent knows that only one tree is off-limits. But he has an agenda, an angle, a thought he desperately needs Eve to adopt. He suggests that what God has prohibited drastically outnumbers what He has permitted for their pleasure and provision. His agenda is to cast even the faintest shadow of doubt in the human psyche toward the Creator and King.

The Serpent referencing "any tree" may seem like a minor detail. Yet if he can convince Adam and Eve that God prohibits more than

He provides, isn't He stingy, unfair, and can't be trusted? If this is a God who won't allow His creation to enjoy fruit from *any* of the trees, isn't His entire character called into question?

The Serpent's goal is for them to entertain doubt-filled thoughts about God:

This is a God who withholds blessing.

This is a God who hides things.

This God doesn't care about us.

This God has secrets.

This is a God of rules.

This God can't provide for our needs.

We can't trust this God; we can trust only ourselves.

Eve responds to the Serpent by declaring that they aren't allowed to even touch the Tree of Knowledge in the middle of the garden. But when did God prohibit *touching* the tree? He didn't. The Mind of Adam will constantly exaggerate God's good rules until they seem illogical and unrealistic.

Adam and Eve begin to wonder about God's character, and the Serpent is still casting doubt on the character and motives of God today. His tricks have never been updated.

What thoughts have you entertained about God? What is your idea of God? What version of God do you believe in?

- Is your version of God holding out on you?
- Is your version of God angry?
- Is your version of God someone you need to fear?
- Is your version of God stingy?
- Is your version of God a dictator?
- Is your version of God the image of your earthly parents?
- Is your version of God making you anxious?

You may have entertained erroneous—heretical—ideas about God, but our first step in redeeming those thoughts is a healthy confrontation of wrong ideas about Him. So let's set a few of them straight.

- God invented sex, so it was His idea.
- God laughs, so He likes fun.
- God made colors and gave us eyes, so He wants us to enjoy them.
- God created taste buds and showed up at weddings with wine.

Any Being who invents sex, laughs, creates colors and taste buds, and provides wine at a wedding seems like a marvelous Being to me. Unfortunately, the Serpent was able to spin a web of deception that caused Adam and Eve to believe that this jovial, loving, and kind God was prohibiting them from enjoying the trees of the garden.

What trees has the Serpent asked you about? What trees do you think God is prohibiting you from enjoying?

- Does your version of God want you poor?
- Does your version of God want you eternally single and celibate?
- Does your version of God want you to be barren?
- Does your version of God want you to be bored?
- Does your version of God want you anxious?

What version of God do you believe in, and which trees is He prohibiting you from enjoying? The God of the Bible provided count- less trees for His children, but He protected them from the one tree He knew was dangerous by saying no. God said yes countless other times. Every loving parent says no when their children are in danger. Good parents don't prohibit sticking items into electrical sockets or running into the street as an expression of hate but rather as an expression of love.

Please allow me to reassure you that . . .

- God is good.
- God is for you, not against you.
- God only wants to protect you.
- God loves you unconditionally.
- God is flawless in His character.
- God is unwavering in His love.
- God is perfect in His judgment.

And because of all these things, you can trust Him.

In his book *The Knowledge of the Holy*, A.W. Tozer writes these three sets of wise words:

> The most portentous fact about any man is not what he at a given time may say or do, but what he in his deep heart conceives God to be like. We tend by a secret law of the soul to move toward our mental image of God.
>
> What comes into our minds when we think about God is the most important thing about us.
>
> Were we able to extract from any man a complete answer to the question, "What comes into your mind when you think about God?" we might predict with certainty the spiritual future of that man.[4]

Tozer communicates all this with a sniper's accuracy, because everything can be traced to our ideas about God. Our ideas about Him will be either poisonous or nutritious to our minds, and an accurate concept of God is the ultimate brain food. Jesus stands at the Tree of Life offering the fruit of orthodox theology. The Serpent still stands at the Tree of Knowledge, offering slanderous half-truths and heresies concerning God.

You can medicate yourself for the rest of your life and still continue to deal with the symptoms of your toxic thoughts, or you can change your mental diet and heal yourself from the inside out. Adam and Eve chose to binge on a diet of doubt and moral independence from the Tree of Knowledge, and until we consume healthy ideas concerning the character of God, we will need to mask our mental pain with various forms of self-medication.

The cross is the Tree of Life, and the cross of Christ is the demonstration of perfect theology. Everything we need to know about God can be clearly seen as Jesus hangs on a tree for the redemption of humanity.

Independence? Or God-Given Ignorance?

When I moved to England years ago, I had an adapter that allowed me to plug my electric shaver into a British outlet. But I hadn't accounted for something. My American shaver vibrated uncontrollably and died because it wasn't built to handle the increased measures of voltage. Similarly, our minds aren't equipped for the knowledge Adam and Eve let leak into the human consciousness, and the Enemy knew this.

The Serpent's sneaky sales pitch to the innocent couple culminated with this statement: "God knows that when you eat from [the tree] your eyes will be opened, and you will be like God, knowing good and evil" (Genesis 3:5). He knew this statement was full of half-truths, hiding dire consequences for both them and for us.

Humans weren't built to handle the knowledge that is destroying us today. We're overinformed. We have access to a level of knowledge that kills—especially now that we're constantly connected to every world crisis through twenty-four-hour news. And though the Serpent told Eve that she and Adam could be like God, we're not gods, and our human frailty is on display, crippling our teenagers with anxiety as the voltage of information tasers them into paralysis.

Adam and Eve's eyes were opened. Because the Serpent introduced distrust for the One who was their moral compass, they chose to be morally independent beings, becoming their own gods. Once there was doubt within the hearts of humans, they dethroned God as the moral lawgiver and bit into the fruit that would make them independent of His moral standard and objectivity.

As long as they trusted and obeyed God by avoiding the Tree of Knowledge of Good and Evil, they were safe as morally dependent beings. Eating from the forbidden tree was the only way to obtain the knowledge of good versus evil. The original design of humanity doesn't include an ability to judge for ourselves what is good and what is evil. Neither has there been an update from the manufacturer. Adam and Eve were sold a lemon. They traded abundant life and unlimited provision for moral independence, because they doubted God's character and motives. And God's crown of moral independence crushed their heads.

The salesman with snakeskin boots, a forked tongue, and greasy slicked-back hair still stands in front of the Tree of Knowledge, offering sons and daughters of Adam and Eve the opportunity to exchange abundant life for moral independence. As we try to escape from God's moral judgment, we run full steam ahead into the pit of confusion, despair, depression, and anxiety. The fruit we stole from the tree of forbidden knowledge is indeed poison.

Anxiety—as well as gender confusion, depression, and every other form of mental unrest—is simply the side effect of wearing God's crown of moral independence. The human soul was designed for moral ignorance, not moral independence.

Maybe it's time to stop eating the forbidden fruit and return to God's throne with His stolen crown, once again becoming loyal, morally dependent beings so we can have true peace of mind. In order for our loving Creator to brain wash our broken minds with the blood of the Lamb, we have to dethrone the false gods of our own opinions and return to dependency on Him alone.

We must accept His verdict regarding what is good.

We must accept His verdict regarding what is evil.

To be dependent on His mind and thoughts alone is to be brain washed. But like our fallen predecessors, we choose to be independent rather than brain washed by a Creator who loves us and knows what's best for us.

We fight it.

We resist it.

We want our opinions.

We want to give the final verdict.

We want the freedom to choose.

We want to choose our gender.

We want to choose our spouse.

We want to define marriage.

We want to be gods.

As long as we enthrone our own opinions, we'll be anxious, depressed, and medicated, and we'll experience mental unrest.

The prophet Isaiah declared that Jesus would be called "Prince of Peace" (Isaiah 9:6). As thousands of people flood into our churches every Sunday, I'm keenly aware that they're looking to Jesus to be their Prince of Peace because they've suffered under the influence of anxiety for so long. Yet it becomes more and more clear that not everyone is willing to make Jesus their Prince. But only when we've made Him the Prince of our lives can He bring us His peace.

So many of us, though—refusing to make Him the Prince of our lives—still ask Jesus for peace that surpasses understanding. Sadly, we're our own "princes." We're filled with anxiety regarding areas of our lives we refuse to place under the lordship of Jesus. We've replaced God's throne with our opinions and feelings, and anxiety proves the experiment has failed. But peace is the exclusive right of those who are actively making Jesus their Prince.

When Jesus is the Prince over our finances, we have financial peace.

When Jesus is the Prince over our marriage, we have marital peace.

When Jesus is the Prince over our career, we have vocational peace.

When Jesus is the Prince over our ministries, we have spiritual peace.

Many of us today are also our own "lords." When my wife and I leased an apartment, we called the landlord whenever something broke or didn't work properly. If the dishwasher malfunctioned or the air conditioning wasn't to our liking, we called the landlord, because the responsibility rests with the owner. But then when we became homeowners, a convenient number to call for help with household maintenance was no longer available. Assuming the role of landlord inevitably came with the responsibility of consistently being the lord of our own land.

When we're the lords of our finances, our marriages, and all our moral decisions, we're inevitably in over our heads. If we want to be our own lords, then we must provide peace, joy, purpose, fulfillment, and mental clarity for ourselves. But the reality is that none of us can do that. We've overplayed our hand.

We aren't good princes; we're inadequate lords. And we aren't competent at playing God's role.

The crown of moral independence has caused a cosmic headache as it rests on the head of humanity, and the sight of our teenagers bent over with anxiety should be a wake-up call for an unconditional surrender.

Based on the name of the forbidden tree, it's clear that God understood how easily thoughts could be weaponized. He allows humanity access to the Tree of Life, and presumptive reasoning would assume that the opposite tree would simply be called the Tree of Death, since eating from it brings death. But God forbids Adam and

Eve to eat from the Tree of Knowledge of Good and Evil because He understands that knowledge isn't always beneficial, and in many cases it kills. The Serpent baits Adam and Eve with a thought, and then they partake of the poisonous fruit of knowledge.

The descendants of Adam and Eve are still dealing with the venomous effects of both.

Anxiety and Grace

Like many people, I've had the awkward privilege of borrowing money from close friends and family members, and nothing has the power to fill the human heart with stress and anxiety like bumping into someone you've borrowed money from before you've had the chance to pay them back. The best-case scenario involves your spotting the person you owe before they spot you, allowing you to control the situation. And yes, by *controlling the situation*, I do mean avoiding that person altogether.

The worst-case scenario is when the cousin-turned-debt-collector startles you in a store's checkout line while you're spending money on something stupid. My hood upbringing may leak through the pages here, but I have seen my fair share of confrontations where the lender demands that items get returned to the shelves. Maybe I'm the only person who's ever heard someone say, "If you got money for Target, you got money to pay me back," but you can put that moment down as one of the top ten embarrassing moments of life.

Regardless of the circumstances, debt brings paranoia. The more debt you have, the more stress and anxiety you feel. At one point, I owed thousands of dollars for parking violations in the state of Massachusetts, and I was paranoid to park because I knew I was at risk of getting a bright-yellow boot placed on the wheel of my car. My friends and I would be downtown, and while they experienced a carefree evening, I'd have this underlying knot of worry playing as background music, coloring my experience.

Inevitably, I was caught. One day I walked out of a shopping center to find my car had been towed to the city impound. But after I paid my debt, I could once again enjoy a stress-free parking experience.

You may not be able to easily draw a straight line between God's grace and your anxiety, but they are directly linked. When you walk through life with this underlying guilt that you're indebted to God, it will inevitably lead to anxiety in your soul. There is no greater peace than knowing that you and God are at peace. Peace with Him creates peace in every other aspect of life. Grace is the understanding that Jesus has paid the debt humanity incurred by eating from the Tree of Knowledge of Good and Evil.

If you believe you owe God,

if you believe He's angry with you,

and if you believe you're in debt to Him,

then you'll avoid Him,

and you'll have this unexplainable anxiety,

and every bad thing that happens you'll consider karma.

But if you know you are debt free,

if you believe God smiles on you,

and if you know there's peace between you and Him,

then your entire life will be filled with peace,

and paranoia and fear will lose their grip on your mind,

and peace with God will produce the peace of God.

This is what I wish I'd said to that anxiety-ridden student in the church lobby.

Drop the Leaves

2

> Then the man and his wife heard the sound of the LORD God as he was walking in the garden in the cool of the day, and they hid from the LORD God among the trees of the garden. But the LORD God called to the man, "Where are you?" He answered, "I heard you in the garden, and I was afraid because I was naked; so I hid."
>
> Genesis 3:8–10

I NERVOUSLY APPROACHED THE DOOR to Dr. Abbott's office building, hoping nobody I knew would spot me. Then I sat in his waiting room while my insecurities tried to convince me that seeing a therapist was unnecessary and I should return to my car and go to work. The last thing I wanted to do was talk to a stranger about the memories I'd successfully managed to suppress for years. To me, talking to a therapist was downright embarrassing and the ultimate display of weakness.

My dad drilled some lessons into me as I was growing up. One was that men never reach into a woman's purse. It is forbidden.

And if a woman asks you to retrieve something from that forbidden purse, you simply hand them the bag.

But more significantly, he drilled these two lessons into my mind and heart:

1. Rules are always optional, and they rarely apply to you. They were created for the people who needed them. (Need I say more?)
2. Don't be weak. We Arangos are strong. Always be strong. If you are indeed hurt or weak, hide it. Pretend to be strong at all costs.

My father demonstrated that last one by shoplifting nice clothes for me. Just because we were poor didn't mean people needed to know it, and of course we wouldn't ask for help when we could break the law to hide our weakness.

You can see why I was so conflicted as I sat in Dr. Abbott's waiting room. Even when you recognize the lessons you learned from your parents are rooted in dysfunction, it is still challenging to completely reject them and break away from their gravitational pull. Those lessons make their way into our minds and souls. I knew Manny Arango Sr. was wrong and insecure, but I couldn't help feeling stupid and silly and uncomfortable that day. I could hear his voice in my head, and I could feel his presence in that waiting room. But I refused to look at Dr. Abbott through the same lens as my dad, so I fought all my natural instincts.

Dr. Abbott finally called me into his office, and we naturally talked about how my dad taught me to never show weakness. At twenty-four years of age, I knew I wasn't weak. But I was broken, confused, angry, and most of all insecure, and I believed my father was the dominant source of my unrest. I had a thorn in my flesh. Even that sounds like an understatement. I had a thorn in my soul.

It's funny how we can be hurt because of someone, but then allow that same person to influence us away from seeking healing. My dad hurt me throughout my childhood and adolescence, and I had almost walked away from a therapist's office because of his continued grip on my mind.

But all things are possible through Christ, and I know I wouldn't have been able to break free in my own power. The Mind of Adam would have kept me bound to the lessons I'd been taught as a child and teenager, but the light of the gospel pierced the dysfunction I was raised in and began to teach me something different. Only the Mind of Christ can do that.

In Paul's second letter to the Corinthian church, he wrote about the thorn in his flesh, openly talking about weakness in a way that would make Manny Arango Sr. cringe.

Therefore, in order to keep me from becoming conceited, I was given a thorn in my flesh, a messenger of Satan, to torment me. Three times I pleaded with the Lord to take it away from me. But he said to me, "My grace is sufficient for you, for my power is made perfect in weakness." Therefore I will boast all the more gladly about my weaknesses, so that Christ's power may rest on me. That is why, for Christ's sake, I delight in weaknesses, in insults, in hardships, in persecutions, in difficulties. For when I am weak, then I am strong (2 Corinthians 12:7–10).

I recall reading that passage for the first time and saying to God, *Paul didn't need Your grace! He needed You to remove the thorn!* I hate looking back on moments when I thought I could offer God wisdom. But in hindsight, I can see I was utterly confused by this passage because I thought God had extended some fuzzy, feel-nice grace when Paul needed rescue. I would soon learn that grace isn't fuzzy at all; it's a force to be reckoned with and a concept that must be grasped if we are to adopt the Mind of Christ.

One fateful Thursday morning, I had a particularly aggravating conversation with Dr. Abbott that radically changed the way I saw both my thorn and Paul's thorn. I had again stealthily entered his building, and as usual I was venting about how terrible my father was. And like always, Dr. Abbott seemed really engaged and entertained by what I was saying, which encouraged me to talk more. (What can I say? I'm a preacher, and I can't resist talking when people want to listen.)

I described my father as manipulative, deceptive, dishonest, and a wordsmith who could talk his way in or out of anything. He was a killer salesman who was charming and charismatic. Even though he battled with a severe drug addiction, he was never unemployed! My dad was a general contractor and could easily talk families into giving him large down payments for jobs and keys to their homes. He was a magician with his words, and I hated him for it.

Dr. Abbott responded that day by saying, "Wow, it sounds like your dad gave you a powerful set of gifts."

In piercing outrage, I responded with one word: "What?"

Dr. Abbott repeated his statement. "Yeah, it sounds like your dad gave you a powerful set of gifts." Then with confidence, he added, "Maybe I missed something. Can you describe him again?"

With a tone of betrayal and aggravation, and filled with an attitude that clapped back at Dr. Abbott, I repeated the list, then ended with, "He did more damage to my mother and me with his words than he ever did with his actions."

With caring eyes and a gentle tone, Dr. Abbott said, "Manny, what do you do for work?"

I told him I was a preacher and a pastor.

"So that means you can talk people out of death and into life, right? That means you're a salesman who can sell abstinence to a teenager, right? Being a preacher means you're a wordsmith. Being a pastor means you need charisma and charm, right? Your father gave you a powerful set of gifts, Manny, and God chose him to be your dad because He knew which raw gifts your destiny would demand."

I couldn't speak. My words were caught in my throat, and tears watered my face. I couldn't stop crying, and I don't even remember how the session ended or walking to my car. But I never snuck into Dr. Abbott's office again. My thorn became my crown. I cried because I had been asking God to remove a thorn, but now I'd finally learned what it felt like to have Him transform a thorn by His grace.

For the first time in my life, I wasn't insecure but rather proud of who my dad was even though the results of his drug addiction had been my biggest insecurity growing up. Every time one of my peers came to church and let me know they'd seen him asking for money on the street, I felt naked and exposed. My pride was desperate for something to cover my nakedness. I made fun of my dad before anyone else could because I was so embarrassed and insecure. I grew up desperately wanting to be a pastor's kid, fantasizing about having a dad who could teach me how to preach. But for starters I just wanted a father I could be proud of.

Yet all along I did have a father who was teaching me how to preach. I just didn't realize it. I didn't need God to remove my thorn; I needed Him to twist it into a crown of dependence on Him. I needed His grace, and as I allowed it to wash my mind and detangle my thoughts, I realized I could have never transformed my mind independent of God's intervention.

My brain was washed that day. I was willing to reject the thought patterns I was taught as a kid, and now God was helping me adopt a new mindset. Insecurity lost its grip, and I would never see or think about my dad the same way.

God's solution regarding our weaknesses is never to remove them but to utilize them, put them on display, and pour His grace out over them. When we're walking in independence from God, our weaknesses inevitably become our insecurities and dominate our thinking. That is the dynamic we observe through the opening pages of

Genesis. Because Adam and Eve chose to act out in independence, they shattered the image of God that gave them confidence and validation. Trapped in insecurity, the young couple became aware of their nakedness and hid.

I believed my dad was the source of all my weaknesses, but the gentle yet powerful force of God's grace, experienced through intimacy, turned my father into the seed of all my strength. It wasn't simply a therapist's tactic that penetrated my heart that day; it was the radical and relentless voice of God that spoke to me through Dr. Abbott.

My prayer is that God will speak to you right now through the pages of this book and that you will be convinced that His grace is sufficient for your weaknesses and insecurities. God can transform your thorns into your crown, so that like Paul, you can declare, "I will boast all the more gladly about my weaknesses, so that Christ's power may rest on me. . . . For when I am weak, then I am strong" (2 Corinthians 12:9–10).

I had always perceived my father as my weakness, and the Mind of Adam taught me to be insecure because of that perceived weakness. God, however, revealed that the problem wasn't my dad but how I thought about him. His drug addiction wasn't the source of my insecurity; the Mind of Adam I used to filter and understand life was the source.

The Mind of Adam is full of insecurity.

Full of embarrassing weaknesses.

Full of hiding.

Full of thorns.

Full of self-pity.

Full of man.

The Mind of Christ is full of identity.

Full of illogical confidence.

Full of vulnerability.

Full of crowns.

Full of power.

Full of God.

We all have insecurities, and when we humans live independently of God, it becomes impossible to keep from drowning in our insecure thoughts. Intimacy with God means we become intimate with grace and our insecurities lose their power. We're still naked, but no longer ashamed.

Adam and Eve had always been naked, but something about the fruit they ate made them aware of their nakedness and embarrassed by it. It wasn't until they chose independence from God that their nakedness became a source of insecurity. The Bible shows us that, after eating the forbidden fruit, Adam and Eve were immediately crippled with insecurity.

Which insecure thoughts have imprisoned you? Maybe, like me, you're insecure about your parents. Maybe you're insecure about your looks. Maybe you're insecure about your past.

As we explore the Mind of Adam, we'll discover the root cause behind our insecure thoughts, and Jesus will equip you to dominate every insecure thought that has plagued you.

Let's keep diving deeper.

Drop the Leaves

We can clearly see how the fruit from the Tree of Knowledge immediately works its debilitating magic. The knowledge of good and evil seems tempting. The initial and lasting side effect of this deadly fruit, however, is insecurity. The fruit is marketed as powerful, but the Serpent knows it's powerfully poisonous for the human soul and psyche. Adam and his bride are immediately afraid, overly aware, and full of shame, and the weight of guilt presses on their sin-sick souls.

Before Adam and Eve's great folly, God had given them an intrinsic understanding of their own value. They walked in the power of self-confidence, and it all flowed from God's truth, not their own opinions. They were created as image-bearers, and therefore possessed a deep and abiding sense of self-worth rooted in God's love for and acceptance of them. This is the mental and emotional state humans were created for and the only state in which we thrive.

Once they were under the influence of sin, Adam and Eve's brilliant plan was to hide from God among the trees and cover their newfound nakedness with fig leaves. Sin immediately made the young couple aware, shameful, and unsafe. The Mind of Adam received an overdose of self-awareness, which always results in shame, insecurity, and fear, causing us to hide from God and others.

We humans have become experts at hiding our flaws and covering up our failures. We descendants of Adam are all keenly aware of our frailties, and we work tirelessly to keep them a secret. But the truth is we're tired. Hiding and covering up our flaws is draining, and Jesus recognized this when He said, "Come to me, all you who are weary and burdened, and I will give you rest. Take my yoke upon you and learn from me, for I am gentle and humble in heart, and you will find rest for your souls. For my yoke is easy and my burden is light" (Matthew 11:28–30).

Genesis 2:25 says, "Adam and his wife were both naked, and they felt no shame," and until humanity adopts the Mind of Christ, we will never rest in the power of that approval again. Notice that when sin was introduced, the couple not only hid from God but from each other. Insecurities not only make intimacy with God impossible but intimacy with others impossible.

The Mind of Christ is God's system for restoring the human soul to factory settings. We were created to flourish in the garden of divine approval and acceptance; adopting the Mind of Christ is not an attempt to discover that approval but to recover it. Until then, our insecurities will place demands for applause on other humans that only God can meet, and we will be continually disappointed in our relationships. Insecurities make humans needy and high maintenance, and relationships that should be loving and peaceful become hard work and a burden.

The depth of a relationship can be measured only by its honesty, and many of us are swimming in the shallow end of relational intimacy because our insecurities prohibit us from launching into the depth of honesty. Without honesty, our insecurities force us to find fig leaves and hide.

What has you wearing fig leaves?

An eating disorder?

A pornography addiction?

An over-reliance on alcohol?

An abuse of prescription drugs?

A cycle of comparison sparked by social media?

Something else that has you bound?

And the Serpent keeps telling you that you can beat this on your own and you don't need help. Maybe you think needing help makes you weak. You're right; it does make you weak. But only when you're weak will God's strength perfect you and His grace be sufficient to cover you.

Whenever we're honest, we remove the fig leaves and are forced to accept our nakedness instead of covering up.

One of the most beautiful Scripture verses is found in God's response to His fig-leaf-covered children. The leaves barely worked to cover their physical nakedness and would always be insufficient to cover their shameful and guilt-ridden souls, so "God made garments of skin for Adam and his wife and clothed them" (Genesis 3:21).

If there were skins, then there was an animal, which means there was a sacrifice, which means there was blood. Adam's guilt and pride turned a dad into a dictator. Adam's guilt and pride were so afraid of being caught that he couldn't foresee that God was there to cover him and Eve, not catch them. The couple saw themselves as criminals, which they were, but God still saw them as His children. God Himself initiates the Old Testament sacrificial system in order to cover Adam and his bride, because "without the shedding of blood there is no forgiveness [of sins]" (Hebrews 9:22).

Adam and Eve covered up their mistake with leaves, but God covered them with blood.

Our loving and gracious Father stands before His delinquent and newly deprived children with grace dripping from His hands in the form of earth's initial bloodshed. Our Father uncovers the flesh of an animal to cover the nakedness of the creatures who bear His image. And in my imagination's eye, Adam and Eve stand there desperately hoping that God will place the freshly skinned furs on top of the already existing fig leaves.

Adam doesn't want to uncover himself in order for God to cover him; that would be even more embarrassing. But he must remove the leaves to receive the skins God has provided. He must return to his state of nakedness for the Father to cover him. The blood can't be applied to the leaves; it must be applied directly to Adam.

Are we really any different from Adam? We want God to heal our brokenness—as long as we don't have to be broken before Him. We want God to cover our nakedness—as long as we don't have to be naked before Him. Adam would love to keep the insufficient fig leaves pressed to his sinful flesh, but God will not have it. Adam's guilt tells him that the Father wants to embarrass him, but truly God's only desire is to empower Adam, because the blood has power only once it's been directly applied to the sinner.

We all have fig leaves that we've sewn together to mitigate our vulnerability, and as long as our trust is in them, we will never be free.

Dad or Dictator?

I'm the first person in my family to graduate from college, so the spring of my senior year was a truly festive and exciting time around the Arango household. My parents wore the pride they had for me on their faces like a new line of cosmetics, and every waiter at every restaurant we visited knew I was soon to graduate from college.

In the midst of all the festivities, my father surprised me with a new car, and I knew for a fact that I had conquered the world. But in gleeful euphoria, I must have mistaken my sporty Honda Civic for a Chevy Tahoe, because it wasn't long before I learned its unique limits. I attempted to drive over a median and got stuck, but I assumed that since I was easily able to be towed and unstuck, no lasting damage was done to the vehicle.

When I parked outside my parents' house that night, though, I noticed the driver's door was slightly ajar because the bottom frame had been bent. I knew my father would be angry, so I had to fix it before he noticed the damage.

A couple of days later, I'd found an auto body technician to do the work, but I didn't have any money to pay for it. So I asked God to make my father distracted, or blind—or anything, really. But I knew that was a long shot. My dad thoroughly inspected my car a couple of times a week, and this week would clearly be no different.

My heart hit my stomach the day I walked into the house and my dad, in the most casual tone ever, asked, "How's your car?"

Immediately sensing he knew the truth, I awkwardly fumbled through my answer. I refused to tell on myself, needing to be caught utterly red-handed before I would divulge any unnecessary information. I acted helplessly oblivious to the damage.

But then my father broke the stalemate of this aggressively casual conversation and said flat out, "I know the frame of your driver's-side door is bent. It looks like your car got stuck on something you tried to drive over." I finally came clean, and my dad told me he had known for days and had already paid someone to fix the door.

Then he asked me a question that hit me as though it were a statement: "Why would you hide this from the only person who would be willing to fix it?" And that day I understood the position Adam and his bride found themselves in as they heard the footsteps of their Creator approaching after their fateful meal near the outlawed tree. I was hiding my car from someone I thought was a dictator ready to catch me. My father wasn't a dictator at all, but my guilt had turned him into one, and my pride told me I could evade his help altogether with my own homemade remedy.

All of us have done the same exact thing to God at some point. Pride can't stand to be bailed out, and it hates handouts and is severely allergic to grace. Guilt always hides from the bright light of truth, and pride always rejects God's charity. Guilt and pride are a deadly combination, and the Mind of Adam is defenseless against both. The Bible teaches that "God opposes the proud but shows favor to the humble" (James 4:6). I wonder if the opposite statement could also be true. Do the proud oppose God? Do the proud oppose grace? My guilt actively worked in opposition against the solution my dad had already prepared and secured. My guilt turned a loving father into a dictator, and I wonder if we do the same with our heavenly Father. Could guilt and pride be the root of all the toxic thoughts running through our minds?

Although God does dictate (we'll talk about that later in the book), He isn't a dictator. He's a dad.

If, like Adam and Eve, we believe God's approaching simply to catch us, we'll cover up. But He never approaches a problem without a solution. Remember, whatever thoughts we have about God determine every other thought we entertain. We are all one heretical thought away from our Jenga tower crashing to the floor.

If God is a dictator, then He can't be trusted, and we must choose independence to provide for ourselves. But choosing independence is sinful, and the image of God in us shatters, the fruit intoxicates us with self-awareness, and self-awareness leads to insecure thoughts. Our independence separates us from God's approval, and we become imprisoned by our own insecure thoughts. They force us to hide from God, and when we hide from Him, we trust Him even less. Then the cycle repeats until a mental loop is fully formed.

As soon as the forbidden fruit dances on the taste buds of humanity, shame is immediately produced, and we reject ourselves because deep within our souls we believe that God has rejected us. God created humans to reflect His glory, so He installed a mirror at the core of our souls. Ideally, when we look in that mirror, we should see the reflection of God. But sin has shattered it, and now every time we look inward, we hate what we see. That broken image is the source of our insecurity.

The mirror hanging on your bedroom wall isn't the source of your insecurity; the one hanging within your soul is the source of your insecurity. You may think you're insecure because of your nose or socioeconomic status or your weight, but those are simply distractions.

Insecurities always turn our gaze and focus inward and allow the ego to take front and center stage of our soul. Much like a flower, the human soul never tends to flourish when it's turned inward on itself. *Insecurity* is simply a euphemism for pride, which is an obsession with self. Whenever the object of our attention is self, we either become overly aware of our imperfections and develop low self-esteem or become overly aware of our gifts and become arrogant.

Unfortunately, many of us have believed that the way to establish confidence is to turn inward and begin to appreciate ourselves, our talents, and the unique qualities we bring to the world. Our value as humans, though, has little to do with who we are and more to do with who created us.

The Adamic approach to building confidence is a fundamentally flawed experiment because humans are sinful. Every son of Adam and every daughter of Eve is born with the shattered glass of God's image at the core. When we look inward to build confidence, we inevitably start looking into the dark depths of our sinful nature, thoughts, habits, and inclinations. To look inward is to look into the mirror that shattered on the day Adam and Eve ate that fateful fruit in the garden. As long as our gaze is inward, we will continue to experience negative side effects, like incessant hiding and the thorns of insecurity.

Where's Your Burning Bush?

Moses—one of the most colorful, dynamic, and iconic characters in the Bible—had a life-altering conversation with God that muted his insecure thoughts and told him his life would never be the same. This trajectory-altering encounter happened when he was an eighty-year-old fugitive, running from the law and living in the wilderness.

God calls out to Moses from a burning bush and tells him He's heard the cry of His enslaved people and has selected him to lead them out of slavery and into a land they will possess as their inheritance. He commands Moses to return to Egypt and declare to Pharaoh that he has been sent by God to declare one message: "Let my people go" (Exodus 8:1).

Moses responds based on the insecure thoughts he's been harboring. He asks two insecure questions followed by two insecure statements:

Moses said to God, "Who am I that I should go to Pharaoh and bring the Israelites out of Egypt?" (Exodus 3:11)

Moses answered, "What if they do not believe me or listen to me and say, 'The LORD did not appear to you'?" (Exodus 4:1)

Moses said to the LORD, "Pardon your servant, Lord. I have never been eloquent, neither in the past nor since you have spoken to your servant. I am slow of speech and tongue." (Exodus 4:10)

Moses said, "Pardon your servant, Lord. Please send someone else." (Exodus 4:13)

Can you hear the paralyzing force of insecure thinking beneath the surface of Moses's words? Can you hear the self-doubt hidden beneath the surface of his inquiry? Moses can't bring himself to believe he's significant, qualified, gifted, respectable, or the right person for the task. He doesn't harbor any negative thoughts about God, but he does harbor negative and insecure thoughts concerning himself.

If Moses was one of your friends and called you to vent about his frustrations regarding this insecurity, you would do what every good friend would do. You'd encourage your good friend Moses by reminding him of his accolades, his education, his giftedness, and his unique ability to lead. Any decent friend would attempt to build his confidence by telling him about himself, by turning his gaze inward.

God, however, understands that would be a practice in futility. He will change Moses's self-deprecating view of himself but not the way one would expect.

God responds to Moses with one statement: "I AM WHO I AM" (Exodus 3:14). He could have spoken to Moses about Moses, but instead, He spoke to Moses about who He was, who He had always been, and who He would always be. God's response to Moses was to reveal to him that confidence doesn't come from within, but rather is revealed from heaven and received through intimacy with God.

Are you battling with insecure thoughts? Then God says to you, *I am who I am.* He doesn't say, *You are who you are.* Confidence is never discovered by looking within. Confidence can only be recovered with God,

revealed by God,

received from God.

By the time Moses confronts Pharaoh, our hero is no longer handicapped by his insecurities and is boldly walking in the miraculous power of God. Moses proves that once we catch a glimpse of God in His glory, we're immediately left with an indelible mark. The thorns of insecure thinking can be transformed into a crown only when we depend on God as the source of our identity. Identity is the fruit of adopting the Mind of Christ. We must, however, continue dismantling the Mind of Adam before we can begin building the Mind of Christ.

We have one more set of ruins to explore in our journey through the Mind of Adam before we can set our sights for the Mind of Christ. We've explored how negative thoughts concerning God will always lead to moral independence followed by anxious thoughts. We've explored how independence from God inevitably leads to an onslaught of insecure thoughts concerning ourselves. Next, we'll explore how insecurities lead to isolation within our interpersonal relationships and how the toxic thoughts associated with how we perceive others can be tamed.

3

Blame Game

The man said, "The woman you put here with me—she gave me some fruit from the tree, and I ate it." Then the LORD God said to the woman, "What is this you have done?" The woman said, "The serpent deceived me, and I ate."

Genesis 3:12–13

A large crowd followed and pressed around him. And a woman was there who had been subject to bleeding for twelve years. She had suffered a great deal under the care of many doctors and had spent all she had, yet instead of getting better she grew worse. When she heard about Jesus, she came up behind him in the crowd and touched his cloak, because she thought, "If I just touch his clothes, I will be healed." Immediately her bleeding stopped and she felt in her body that she was freed from her suffering.

At once Jesus realized that power had gone out from him. He turned around in the crowd and asked, "Who touched my clothes?"

Mark 5:24–30

I'M A HUGE FAN of the TV show *Breaking Bad*. I've watched the entire series from pilot to finale three times, and I even nerd out to YouTube videos explaining its cinematography and character development. So naturally, when a church in New Mexico wanted me to preach for them, I jumped at the opportunity. *Breaking Bad* was filmed in Albuquerque, New Mexico, and I figured I could easily pay homage to Jesus by preaching the gospel and pay homage to the most loved villain of my lifetime—Walter White—on the same trip.

Although all the places I wanted to visit have different names in real life, I planned out a tour to relive my favorite moments from the show. I knew the exact angle I'd use to snap a photo of myself in front of the Crystal Palace and which meal I'd order at Los Pollos Hermanos. At my request, my host from the church even ran his car through the A1A Car Wash where Walter laundered his drug money.

The crown jewel of my *Breaking Bad* tour was the house portrayed as Walter and Skyler White's home. As soon as we turned onto the street, my mind was flooded with memories from the show. The iconic residence was the epicenter of Walter White's family drama, and I felt emotionally connected to the place. I remembered when Holly was brought to this home and placed in her crib. I remembered the sound of Walt Jr.'s crutches as he walked down the hallway. I remembered the first time Walt shaved his head in the bathroom sink of the master suite and in exactly which walls he had his money hidden. I remembered the conversations in the kitchen and the stuffed animal that fell from the sky and landed in Walt's pool.

As soon as we arrived at the house, however, I knew something wasn't quite right. For starters, in the show the home didn't have a huge, fortress-looking wrought-iron fence guarding the unassuming and humble property. Second, it had no sign informing fans and tourists to "Take Your Pictures from Across the Street." Last, in the show no cranky older couple sat on the front lawn yelling at people.

Yup, you read that correctly. As soon as we pulled around to the other side of the street and entered a line of vehicles with people all waiting to snap photos, we realized that the couple who live in the house were sitting on the front lawn barking at every fan who wanted to pay homage to Heisenberg, Walter's alias.

I'm sad to admit that my visit to what fans know as 308 Negra Arroyo Lane was less than magical. Walter White's infamous residence reportedly receives more than a hundred tourists a week, and it became abundantly clear that they're all unwanted guests.

To my mind, the disenfranchised homeowners had eagerly accepted the leading roles the Serpent would love all of us to play—eternal victims. Every tourist who drove past the house was an evil villain, and they were the sad victims who desperately wanted to be left alone. They'd never owned up to the chancy decision they'd made to rent their home to a TV production crew, and the blame for their perpetual dismay at the outcome fell like an avalanche on every fan who approached the house.

Once we adopt a victim mentality, our perspective is poisoned, and the lens we view life through is discolored and distorted. Victim mentality receives information only through the eyes of bitterness.

Adam and Eve are immediately stuck in victim mentality once God confronts them regarding their sin. Adam blames Eve because he's too insecure to do otherwise. Eve points her finger directly at the Serpent. Neither takes responsibility for the part they played, because the only part the Mind of Adam ever chooses to play is the part of the victim in life's unfolding drama. To have the Mind of Adam is to live in an eternal state of victimhood and bitterness.

We could argue that the blame game is quite literally the oldest game on the planet, but to adopt the Mind of Christ is to utterly reject all requests to join in on the game that never has a victor. Only villains and victims are allowed to play the blame game, so our victorious Savior and those who follow Him are excluded from playing.

The Serpent's final goal for humankind was isolation from one another, and he played his hand masterfully. Humans are communal in nature and were designed for interdependent relationship. Once Adam blamed Eve for their sin, the Serpent knew the last domino had fallen. Adam and Eve chose independence over intimacy; insecurity followed, and now the Serpent had successfully forced the man and the woman into isolation as they both played the victim card in their relative corners of self-inflicted solitary confinement.

The Mind of Adam lives in moral independence.

The Mind of Adam is poisoned by insecurity.

The Mind of Adam starves in isolation.

Victim mentality and a bitter perspective mark the Mind of Adam as humanity was tricked into isolation by the deception of the Serpent, whose tactic was to divide and conquer.

Not much has changed.

I don't know all their circumstances, of course (and in their defense, by all accounts the fence went up to keep pizzas off the roof—see the second episode of the third *Breaking Bad* season), but I couldn't help but judge the residents of Walter and Skyler's famed home a little. They clearly saw the property as a burden, whereas I saw it as a possible gold mine. My entrepreneurial mind immediately conjured up business ideas that might even allow the grumpy owners to buy a new home in a nicer part of town. I couldn't believe they were so bitter at the possible source of a blessing. But they seemed to have adopted thought patterns of victimhood and perspectives of bitterness that clouded their perspective on the matter, and that's unfortunate, because mindset and perspective are everything. The owners saw themselves as unlucky victims, and the Mind of Adam can never be towed out from the mental ditch of victim mentality.

Have you barked at blessings because of your bitterness?

Do your defense mechanisms keep you isolated?

Have your insecurities sabotaged your opportunities?

Has playing the blame game cost you relationships?

Have you cast yourself as a perpetual victim?

If so, this chapter is for you.

New Eyes

In Matthew 6:22–23, Jesus says "the eye is the lamp of the body. If your eyes are healthy, your whole body will be full of light. But if your eyes are unhealthy, your whole body will be full of darkness. If then the light within you is darkness, how great is that darkness!" Jesus is teaching that there's an important relationship between your eyes and your mind.

Anyone who passed eighth-grade science knows that our eyes receive information and then feed that information to our brain. When we adopt the Mind of Adam, we're constantly taking in information with a lens of victimization. Adopting the Mind of Christ requires a change of perspective on life so we can recognize opportunity and blessing when they are presented. Simply put, the Mind of Christ requires that we also adopt the eyes of faith, gratitude, and victory. Adam is the archetype for victimhood, whereas Christ is eternally victorious. Much like the disgruntled residents of the *Breaking Bad* house seemed to me, many of us kill opportunities for blessing because we can't see our lives properly.

Perspective is essential because God never places blessing in our hands; He places blessing within our reach. God never delivers a final product to our doorstep; He places blessing in our lives in seed form. And seeds are difficult to discern. Blessing is always camouflaged, using the gift-wrapping paper of hard work, transformation, and discipline. We throw away seeds and then wonder why we're fruitless. I was bitter at my father for being a drug addict, but then a therapist helped me clearly see that my dad gave me all the seeds I needed to produce a harvest of blessing in my life. In my bitterness I misjudged my father, because bitterness always ruins our perspective and damages our lens of clarity.

A quick trip to a Walmart superstore will show you that seeds look nothing like the fruit they produce. Watermelon seeds are not green with long stripes, and banana seeds aren't yellow or curved. In the same way, the seeds of peace may not always look like you suspected they would, and the seeds necessary to produce joy in your life may not look the way you expected. Sometimes the business idea that could bring your family wealth may appear in the seed form of annoying tourists, or the King of the world may appear in the seed form of a baby in a manger.

The Mind of Christ gives us new perspective so we can overcome bitterness and doubt and stop throwing away the seeds of power, purpose, and destiny.

Because She Thought

The fifth chapter of Mark's Gospel tells us about a woman who had legitimate reasons to be doubtful and bitter. She had every right to be depressed and every excuse to complain. Her life warranted the adoption of victim mentality, and she had every opportunity to entertain toxic thoughts.

We're introduced to her as Jesus is following Jairus, the ruler of the local synagogue. The Bible explains that the woman had a non-stop flow of menstrual blood that prohibited her from participating in any religious activities in Israel. The Old Testament is clear that when a woman was experiencing her monthly cycle, she was to remain isolated because ceremonial uncleanness could be transferred by touching. The Old Testament gives details concerning the uncleanness of the situation. It says if a woman sat on a piece of furniture while experiencing her monthly cycle, the furniture became unclean, and the next person to sit on it was unclean as well and couldn't participate in the worship of Israel's God.

This woman's medical issue kept her from getting married or having children. Every couple of months a new doctor would tell her about some treatment that would cure her, and in high hopes she would spend money only to find she was sold a box of empty promises. She was isolated. She was an outcast living in chronic discomfort. She spent a fortune on bogus cures. She was known in public by the most private of problems. She was unmarried and barren.

This woman would never know the joy of being held by a lover or the frustration of planning a wedding. And if she were with us today, under the same rules, she would never eat in a restaurant. She'd never sit on a friend's couch, because then the next person to sit on it would be considered unclean.

This woman was socially, physically, and financially down-and-out, but somehow she was mentally, spiritually, and emotionally strong and healthy. Even though her hopes had been high before, only to crash into reality as doctors sold her empty promises, she still had the mental clarity to believe that Jesus could be her solution.

The Bible says, "She came up behind [Jesus] in the crowd and touched his cloak, because she thought, 'If I just touch his clothes, I will be healed'" (Mark 5:27–28).

Because she thought.

Those three words.

Full of power.

This book's entire message could be summed up in those three words. *Because she thought.* (Or because *he* thought.) This woman was healed because of how and what she thought. She was brain washed. She teaches us that our circumstances don't dictate our thoughts; our thoughts determine everything about our lives. Our minds and our perspectives are the control centers of our lives, and everything from our feelings to our finances flows from the health or the poison of our mind's eye. Unbeknownst to this unnamed woman, she was one thought away from the power of miraculous healing flowing through her entire body.

One thought away.

Those three words.

Full of power.

You may also be one idea away. One idea away from seizing breakthrough or encountering healing. You may be one idea away from choosing sobriety or building generational wealth. You could be one idea away from adopting the Mind of Christ.

Like the unnamed woman, we are always one thought away. It's tempting to focus on her touch that brought healing into her life. Indeed, she touched the hem of Jesus's cloak and received healing. But without the correct thought, there would never have been the correct touch. The disciples acknowledged that many people touched Jesus that day, but what sets this woman apart is the thought that preceded her touch.

Much like the residents of Walter White's house did at the sight of tourists, I would have probably approached Jesus with barking as opposed to reaching out in faith after twelve long years of pain, disappointment, and isolation. Bitterness would have potentially pushed me to approach Him with a complaint or to vent and voice my frustrations. Twelve years is a long time to be stuck in physical sickness and seemingly abandoned by God. Two years may not spark frustration and disappointment. Five years may not lead to total discouragement. But twelve years of suffering may spark bitterness in the heart of the most optimistic Christian, and I can imagine that if I had been in this woman's shoes, I might have approached Jesus with a slight attitude.

To be completely honest, I've never waited twelve years for anything, yet I've still grown frustrated and disappointed with God. I've complained after twelve *months* of waiting for Him to work a miracle. But this woman who had been identified by her private pain for a dozen years approached Jesus full of faith and humility.

Her thinking informed and guided her approach as well as her posture, and we must study both to adopt the Mind of Christ.

When our perspective is off and our lens of faith is damaged, we aren't able to see ourselves properly. The woman doesn't approach Jesus as a victim because she doesn't believe she *is* a victim. I've learned that I can receive pity or power from Jesus, but I can't receive them at the same time. The woman had not been pitying herself, so therefore she didn't place a demand on Jesus to pity her. She realized that something far more valuable than pity was available to her—the miraculous and freeing power of Jesus—and she dared not waste her opportunity by filling His ears with a pitiful play-by-play of her twelve years of pain. This woman didn't want pity but power.

The Mind of Adam seeks pity and sympathy.

The Mind of Christ is full of power and strength.

When we adopt the Mind of Christ, we begin to recite the soliloquy of the silent, and the lines we rehearse in our minds become full of positivity and power.

The inner dialogue of your soul will dictate what you verbally declare when given the chance to speak. I'm impressed by this woman because she uses no words, yet her action reveals that her silent soliloquy is full of faith and informed by a healthy perspective. And her posture? The woman doesn't have an entitled posture. She isn't full of pride. She dares not talk to Jesus face-to-face.

When God's timing or inaction disappoints us, we can become like spoiled children throwing a temper tantrum in front of our parents while standing in the very house they've provided for us. This woman's humility is an indictment on an entitled generation infatuated with instant reward and gratification. She crawls to Jesus on her hands and knees in humble worship. Her posture is one of humility, worship, and adoration.

When we focus our attention on our wounds, however, we're filled with resentment and regret, and we withhold worship. Yet worship has the ability to fix our perspective. In worship we forget our wounds as we begin to survey the wounds of our Savior, and we find healing.

When I look at the wounds inflicted on Christ, I realize I don't even deserve to live. I don't deserve the breath in my lungs. Even in our suffering we must approach Jesus with gratitude and worship because of the salvation His wounds have procured on our behalf. We can't be so focused on what God hasn't done that we refuse to worship Him for what He *has* done.

What caused this woman to worship? Her perspective. She approached Jesus because she knew how to discern the mysterious hand of God that sustains us through the storms of life. Life may not be perfect, but as long as there's breath in our lungs, God deserves our allegiance. Sometimes He doesn't heal our lives, but He sustains them, and for His sustaining power over us He is worthy of praise.

The Mind of Adam is entitled and ungrateful. It has eyes that fixate only on disappointment and failed expectations. But the Mind of Christ has a perspective on pain that sets Christianity apart. This impressively powerful woman wasn't *suffering* with a blood issue. This mentally tough champion was *surviving* with a blood issue.

The Mind of Adam naturally counts the years of suffering, but the Mind of Christ automatically counts the years of surviving.

We are survivors.

Those three words.

Full of power.

You survived the cancer.

You survived the divorce.

You survived the abuse.

You survived the layoffs.

You survived the foreclosure.

You survived the addiction.

You survived the depression.

You survived the unbelief.

You survived, and now you're just one thought away.

Victims suffer.

Victors survive.

Bitterness will immediately cause you to identify areas where you've suffered. Jesus doesn't discount or disregard our suffering; He simply helps us see our suffering clearly, in proper perspective, through healthy eyes. Although you've suffered, your pain doesn't have to define your season. The Mind of Christ fixes our perspective. The Mind of Christ writes the mental script we rehearse in the privacy of our thoughts.

And the Mind of Christ always restores identity. That's why Jesus declares publicly who this woman is: "Daughter, your faith has healed you" (Mark 5:34). She is a daughter of God.

The Man by the Pool

For perspective's sake, the unnamed woman from Mark chapter 5 must be seen in contrast to the paralyzed man in John chapter 5. John recounts that Jesus visited the pool of Bethesda and encountered a man who had been paralyzed for thirty-eight years. John 5:6 says that "when Jesus saw him lying there and learned that he had been in this condition for a long time, he asked him, 'Do you want to get well?'"

The Mind of Christ is on full display with this one question. I have had the pleasure of visiting the exact spot where the miracle of this man's healing occurred, and I learned that paralyzed people were placed at this pool because of its prime location. The pool was perfectly positioned for garnering pity and sympathy from the droves of people who had to walk past it to get to their destinations. Jesus asks the man if he wants to get well because healing won't be conducive to his current lifestyle. Healing may actually be disruptive to his modus operandi. He's been placed at the perfect location to garner pity from passersby and has made a living doing so for thirty-eight years, but begging for money will no longer be appropriate or possible once he's healed.

Jesus gives this man the same choice He gives the unnamed woman and all of us—the choice between pity and power, between sympathy and strength.

Healing will remove his victimhood.

Healing will mean he must get a job.

Healing will eliminate the pity parties.

Healing will require newfound responsibility.

Healing isn't always convenient.

The Mind of Christ brings healing, and Jesus will never force us into a new way of life. He wants us aware of the responsibility that accompanies healing. There's still time to wallow in pity if that's what you really want, but rejecting the Mind of Adam will remove the comfortable excuses you may have grown accustomed to.

Adopting the Mind of Christ removes victimhood.

Adopting the Mind of Christ comes with responsibility.

Adopting the Mind of Christ isn't always convenient.

Jesus's question is met with a rather interesting answer. The man replies, "I have no one to help me into the pool when the water is stirred. While I am trying to get in, someone else goes down ahead of me" (John 5:7). In contrast to the unnamed woman who silently approached Jesus, this paralyzed man would rather be heard than healed. He unfortunately has a sad soliloquy that he's eager to share with anyone who will listen. A simple yes would have sufficed as a solid answer to Jesus's inquiry, but when people have adopted an identity of victimhood, they spew resentment all over their listeners, and they bark at their blessings. This man has mentally rehearsed his response to Jesus, and the moment he's given an opportunity, he begins to recite the soliloquy of the sad.

Yet the paralyzed man says enough to communicate that he does in fact possess faith. He doesn't have faith in Jesus, but he certainly has faith in the power of the pool. Jesus takes the man's misplaced faith and redirects its power by healing him and proving that the Son of Man is greater than any pool.

Remember, the Mind of Christ is constantly at work to redeem three categories of thoughts:

1. Thoughts about God
2. Thoughts about self
3. Thoughts about others

Therefore, throughout the pages of the New Testament, Jesus Christ is on a mission to reverse the effects of the fall with new mindsets of wholeness and harmony. The woman touches God wrapped in flesh, and that touch represents that Jesus broke the human cycle of independence. The woman receives healing, making her whole again, so that her physical state is no longer inconsistent with her mental and emotional state. The healing represents the inner healing of cohesion that occurs when our spirit, soul, mind, and body are not at war against one another.

Last, Jesus reconnects the two main characters of the story, which represents the end of human division and isolation. From the outside looking in, it's plausible to assume that Jairus and this unnamed woman have nothing in common.

Jairus is a religious leader.
Jairus is well known and socially connected.
Jairus has financial means.

The woman is a religious outcast.
The woman is known by her issue and is disconnected.
The woman has spent all she has.

Yet Mark weaves their stories together like the writers for TV's *This Is Us*. The very year the woman became ill, Jairus's daughter was born. While there would have been mourning in one doctor's office, there would have been great rejoicing in the other. Their paths cross as they both have needs only Jesus can meet.

Jairus approaches Jesus first and asks if He will come to his house and heal his daughter. But while Jesus is headed to Jairus's house, our unnamed woman reaches out to grab His clothes, and a conversation ensues. Jairus must have been scared and angry as he could see the sand of his daughter's life slipping through the hourglass of time.

The miracle of this story is in the conversation, even though it could cost the girl her life and Jairus the joys of fatherhood. It must be incredibly relevant and pertinent if Jesus feels comfortable allowing a girl the age of a middle school student to die rather than interrupt His communicating with this woman. The conversation is even intentionally within earshot of Jairus, because Jesus meant for him to overhear it: "Daughter, your faith has healed you. Go in peace and be freed from your suffering" (Mark 5:34).

Where the collective soul of society bends toward separation and isolation, Jesus actively works to build unity and connection.

He wanted to teach Jairus a lesson about community, family, and isolation, and He still wants to teach humanity a lesson about how connected our lives really are.

Like many of us would, Jairus identifies his biological daughter as his priority. But Jesus brings a subtle challenge and identifies the woman as a daughter as well and therefore an equal priority. Without question, Jairus would have been the religious leader responsible for isolating this woman and ensuring that she didn't spread her uncleanness to the community. But he would have simply been doing his religious duty, because religion always isolates people with problems. Jesus wasn't a religious leader, though, so He didn't isolate the woman but called her "daughter" and reestablished her status within that community.

Jesus simply calling the woman "daughter" challenged Jairus's worldview, and it challenges ours as well. With one statement Jesus declared that Jairus should see this woman as an irreplaceable part of the community. She had been treated like a problem to manage instead of a person to love, and Jesus prioritizes the confrontation of our toxic thoughts toward one another. He declares that nobody is dispensable and that we are all interconnected and beautifully interdependent.

This story about the woman, before Jesus goes on to raise Jairus's daughter from the dead, doesn't simply end with healing but with the reversal of the Serpent's ploy to divide and conquer. It ends with her reentering the community. She took a risk by rebelling against Jairus's rule to stay isolated, and human touch healed her. Jesus fights for the radical restoration of human connection that Adam and Eve enjoyed in the garden before there was ever insecurity, blaming, and bitterness.

Jairus cared about his daughter, and Jesus had a daughter whom He wanted Jairus to care for as well. Humanity is naturally bent toward isolation and separation, but Jesus made Jairus aware of the complex interconnectedness of life and the interdependence of human life. Human connection brought healing to the woman, and human connection is what Jesus calls all of humanity toward.

How are human connection and our thoughts related?

I'm glad you asked.

Snuggle Service

I thought my friend was joking when he told me he was considering a part-time job as a professional snuggler. But then he showed me a website where you could either train to become certified as a snuggler or enter your credit card information to have a snuggler dispatched to your residence. If you think I'm kidding, please stop reading and search the internet for "snuggle services."

As soon as I saw the website, I was confronted with the sad reality that, as a society, we're splintered, separated, and desperate for intimacy social media has not brought. In fact, we're so desperate for human touch and relationship that some of us are willing to pay strangers by the hour to come to our homes and snuggle with us. Our insecurities keep us in hiding, and the blame game brings more and more division.

Our society is full of disconnected individuals who are suffering mentally from addiction, anxiety, depression, and other toxic mindsets. But many of our mental strongholds could be broken by the power of authentic community and connection. Solitary confinement causes prisoners to lose their mental bearings, and our current trends are becoming more and more socially confined and isolated. Yet we're confused about why we're losing our mental bearings.

Jesus intentionally prolongs a conversation with a newly healed woman so she and Jairus can have a shot at community, family, and love. Adopting the Mind of Christ is a personal journey, but it's not a private journey. As we approach Jesus for mental healing, He will always be standing there ready to connect us with others with whom we didn't think we had anything in common.

4

Just Talking?

... to make her holy, cleansing her by the washing with water
through the word . . .

Ephesians 5:26

The word of God is alive and active. Sharper than any double-edged
sword, it penetrates even to dividing soul and spirit, joints and
marrow; it judges the thoughts and attitudes of the heart.

Hebrews 4:12

I HAD SUCCESSFULLY MANAGED to keep my virginity until my
fateful freshman year of college, and then the pleasure of the moment quickly faded as fear formed a knot in my stomach and kept
me awake at night. I was convinced the girl I was seeing and I
were pregnant and I would have to drop out of college and work at
Starbucks to support a family.

If you've ever had a pregnancy scare, you know firsthand that it's
worse than any roller coaster, haunted house, or suspense thriller
combined. You pray. You call friends. You promise God to never

even kiss again. And you're in a constant state of vigilant expectation for the verdict that will determine the rest of your life.

Thankfully, I was relieved to learn that I didn't have to drop out of college, and the knot finally dissipated. In the coming months, however, I learned that an invisible conception had certainly taken place within my soul.

Intimacy doesn't always lead to a physical pregnancy, but a hundred percent of the time intimacy does lead to the impregnation of ideas, feelings, and soul ties for each person involved. There is no protection against the invisible impregnation that inevitably follows when intimacy occurs between two people.

For months after losing my virginity, I struggled with anger for the first time in my life. I had never had a temper, but I kept experiencing outbreaks of anger and rage. I was utterly confused as to why I was acting so out of character, and then a light bulb went on. The girl I was intimate with had a terrible temper, and emotions as well as ideas and habits are the fruit of our intimate relationships.

Maybe, like me, you've been relieved once or twice at the news that you weren't about to become a parent. The relief is truly short-lived, though, because as I said, although there may not be a physical pregnancy, you are certainly still pregnant.

Many of us are pregnant with insecurities, doubts, and fears. Others of us are pregnant with anxiety, depression, and rage. In the same way that seeds have the power to create new life, words have the ability to create our invisible worlds.

This explains why Jesus describes the Word of God as seed in Luke 8:11. In the same way that physical seeds lead to natural conception and eventual birth, the invisible seeds planted within our souls during intimate moments create conception within our soul and spirit. The Serpent correctly discerned that God's intimacy with humanity was a threat, and he was wise to sever the connection before the seeds of God's Word could blossom and give birth to godly ideas within the souls of Adam and Eve. The Serpent used the power of intimacy to sow seeds of independence in their minds.

The ultimate question of life is whether you will allow the Serpent to plant seeds in the soil of your mind or allow God to plant seeds there. And the question isn't whether your brain is washed. As I said earlier, everyone's brain is—either by the Serpent or by our Creator.

All your relationships can be divided into those two neat categories. Your friends, classmates, and coworkers are either sowing the seeds of God-ideas or sowing the seeds of the Serpent. And since humans are wired for intimacy and crave intimate relationships, we're typically unaware of the cross-pollination of ideas taking place all around us.

Jesus found Himself in this exact scenario with His friend and follower Peter. Jesus pulled together His most intimate inner circle and explained that He would soon die and be raised to life three days later. Peter was not having it, though. Matthew 16:22 says he "took [Jesus] aside and began to rebuke him. 'Never, Lord!' he said. 'This shall never happen to you!'"

Before we examine Jesus's response to Peter, let me remind you that for the three years leading up to this conversation, Peter had been with Jesus every day. They'd shared meals together, they'd walked on water together, and they'd traveled the entire countryside of Israel together. If that doesn't prove the intimacy level of this relationship to you, allow me to remind you that Jesus was so intimate with Peter that He was invited to meet Peter's mother-in-law. Meeting an in-law is one step away from free access to the refrigerator.

Verse 23 informs us that "Jesus turned and said to Peter, 'Get behind me, Satan! You are a stumbling block to me; you do not have in mind the concerns of God, but merely human concerns.'"

Wow! Ouch. I've been called some hurtful names. Unlike Peter, though, I have never been called Satan. You may find Jesus's response to be extreme, but I think He understands something that goes undetected and untraced by most people: Words are never *just* words but seeds, and the people closest to you have the power to plant seeds quicker and deeper than anyone else. Jesus identified the source of Peter's words as satanic because only two factories produce the seeds of ideas. At any given moment we're planting or receiving either the seeds of a God-idea or the Serpent's chosen idea for our downfall and destruction.

Jesus wasn't going to allow Peter to plant the Serpent's seed into His mind. He discerned that in that moment, Peter was recklessly scattering seed from the wrong bag and being used as an agent of Satan to distract and deter Jesus from His purpose. So Jesus took responsibility to protect the soil of His mind. We must do the same if we're to adopt the Mind of Christ.

The Serpent entered Adam and Eve's intimate garden space to introduce an idea that caused them to choose independence, lose their identity, and isolate. But new ideas about God have the power to help us reestablish intimacy with Him. Then as a result of that intimacy, God begins to plant the seeds of identity within our souls, making interdependent relationships possible. Thus far on our journey, we've been learning from Adam's mistake, but this chapter marks a shift where we'll begin to discover Jesus's model.

Adam's mistake is outlined as the threefold descent of independence, insecurity, and isolation. Jesus's model is built based on the blueprint of intimacy, identity, and interdependence. Now let's discover Jesus's model for intimacy and how this foundational step is the catalyst we need for cultivating the Mind of Christ within us.

In chapter 2 of this book, we discovered that the Serpent was able to attack Adam and Eve's intimate relationship with their Creator and King by planting the seeds of doubt-filled ideas, and we studied how intimacy was broken based on ideas. In this chapter we'll discover how the right ideas can flourish based on the soil of healthy intimacy. Our intimate relationships are the most accurate predictors of the ideas that will influence our lives.

Who Told You That?

Adam and Eve's nude streak came to a screeching halt as God descended the heavenly staircase, calling for His wayward honeymooners. Paradise was short-lived as Adam and God entered into an eye-opening conversation that will ultimately help us on our journey.

> The LORD God called to the man, "Where are you?" He answered, "I heard you in the garden, and I was afraid because I was naked; so I hid." And [God] said, *"Who told you that you were naked?* Have you eaten from the tree that I commanded you not to eat from?" (Genesis 3:9–11, emphasis mine)

Adam tells God about his fear, his nakedness, and his decision to hide. God's immediate response is the door this chapter will hinge on. God's answer to Adam's fear and nakedness had nothing to do with either fear or nakedness but with intimacy and influence.

God answers by asking, "Who told you that?" He examines the crime scene with forensic expertise and immediately detects the presence and power of intimacy. Adam's mind has been tampered with by an outside influence, and God knows ideas are born out of an intimate conversation. Ideas can move only through the door of influence, which is securely hinged on the frame of intimacy.

The more intimate a relationship becomes, the more influence the relationship carries. That means the easier ideas can pass between parties, and ideas travel in the vehicle of words and communication. If we're to take our ideas seriously and have brains washed in the blood of Christ, then we'll have to take an inventory of the intimate relationships in our lives. That's because intimacy determines ideas. Our ideas will always be influenced by those with whom we are in intimate relationship, and we have the power to move the mountains of ideas by properly using the lever of intimacy.

The Serpent's well-crafted temptation had a chance of working only if he could get within earshot of the inexperienced and naïve couple. He formed a brilliant idea, but that would prove insignificant if he couldn't influence humanity with it. The Serpent's idea was dependent on whether the couple would choose to entertain the conversation.

He enters their intimate space and sows an idea that causes them to break their intimate ties with their God and choose independence instead. In one fell swoop the Serpent swings the momentum of all creation and turns the tide of the cosmic war for the colony of Earth. He understands that when the tide of intimacy turns, the tide of ideas follows quickly behind. The two tides are tethered together. But we're going to use this timeless truth to our advantage. Based on the beautiful and orthodox ideas we've learned about our gracious and fun-loving God, we'll reestablish intimacy with Him so He can turn the tide of our wild thoughts and calm the storms of our raging souls.

If you feel hopeless in the battle over your mind, I promise that this first step will lead to freedom. Stop thinking about your thoughts and monitoring your ideas. Instead of controlling ideas, control the gates of influence that rest on the hinges of intimacy. You will begin to realize that the light of God's truth has always been there but wasn't visible because of the mental fog and cloud of pollution deposited by others. We all have people in our lives who need to be addressed by the role they're playing and the seeds they're holding.

So many of us attend church on Sundays, where the soil of our minds receive the seeds of God-thoughts. But then for the remainder of the week, the Serpent plants toxic weeds to grow alongside the fruit of the Spirit. In order to walk in the clarity of thought God has for you, two "farmers" can't continue to plant opposing seeds in the field of your mind.

God asks Adam, "Who told you that you were naked?" This can better be translated as . . .

"Who have you been talking to?"

"Who's been in your ear?"

"Who gave you that advice?"

"Who have you been hanging out with?"

"Who have you been intimate with?"

"Who impregnated you with that thought?"

Conversation is an intensely intimate act. Many of the young adults at my church would downplay the true power of conversation by saying things like, "Well, Pastor Manny, we're just talking."

Just talking.

Adam and Eve were *just* talking to the Serpent. The Bible never records that Samson had sex with Delilah; they were *just* talking, and it cost Samson his strength and life. Prayer is *just* talking. When God created the world, He was *just* talking. Maybe talking is the engine that drives intimacy. Maybe talking opens the gates to our souls and allows other people's ideas to infiltrate the motherboard of the brain God is trying to wash.

My hunch is that if you start talking to God, His ideas will populate your world and your mind. I have another hunch. If you start talking to people who talk to God, who are wise and full of faith, more of the ideas you want will crowd out the ideas you've been trying to evict. I firmly believe that if you become intimate with the Mind of Christ and the body of Christ, the ideas of Christ will begin to permeate and protect your mind.

Conversely, I have a hunch that if you continue to keep an open-door policy with toxic people who spew bitterness and doubt, who gossip and complain and talk negatively, their ideas will inevitably color your world.

I have always wondered why God caused the Serpent to crawl on his belly as his just punishment for tricking our vulnerable fore-parents. My holy imagination wonders if the punishment was God's attempt to create distance between the Serpent's slithering tongue and our itching ears.

This chapter is about reclaiming your intimate spaces so you can reestablish intimacy with God, all so your mind can be impregnated with the right ideas.

Pinky and the Brain

It's so fascinating *and* frustrating that most of our insecurities are typically triggered by some sort of comparison with others.

I had no clue I was vertically challenged until my first day of elementary school, but my ignorance was the result of not having had classmates before. My mom had meticulously homeschooled me until the first grade, and I was mentally sharp but completely unaware of my chronic height deficit disorder.

But being short isn't an intrinsic quality, so it can be observed only via comparison. I was short only because I was short*er* than my classmates, and after the first couple of weeks at school, I felt completely betrayed by my parents for keeping me in the dark regarding my height disadvantage. Certainly they could have prepared me for the constant barrage of short jokes and the well-meaning but condescending statements from adult faculty and staff.

Eventually, the elastic band of my confidence snapped, and in anger, I accused my parents of lying to me and blamed them for the height deficit my classmates had diagnosed. Once puberty hit and Sex Ed became a required class, I learned that my indictment of them was scientifically accurate, but that's totally beside the point.

My dad responded by asking me a poignant and pivotal question. With God-like authority, he said, "Who told you that you were short?" My newfound ideas had set off his alarm for new intimate relationships and influences in my life.

In the same way God asked Adam and Eve who told them they were naked, my father didn't deny the validity of my claim but denied the validity of the information's source. He wanted to know whose ideas were running rogue through his son's mind. He wanted to track the footprints and run the forensics on the idea in the hopes that the evidence would lead him to a suspect whose influence had corrupted my mind.

By no means was my father perfect. Yet when it came to this area of my life, he was an absolute hero. He had a keen awareness and an acute understanding that, although the kids at school could and would freely offer their opinions about his son, he was the only man with the authority to speak identity over my life. My classmates had their opinion, but their opinion couldn't compare to the authority of my father's voice.

We can't think about the word *authority* without considering its relation to the word *author*. My father was the author of my life, which gave him unique authority to speak concerning my identity. He took his rightful place as the protector of my forming and fledgling sense of self. He took responsibility for understanding my insecurities and shaping my identity. He understood that I was his son and that children have a reserved and circumspect ear to hear the voice of approval, validation, and identity coming from their dads.

Unfortunately, I encounter a plethora of dads who are either silent or critical of their children, not realizing the weight their voice carries in the souls of their sons and daughters. Somehow, my dad's radar was sensitive to my insecurities, and he took advantage of everyday experiences to create confidence and identity in my soul.

Like most lazy Saturday mornings, I slept to my heart's content and then replaced the daily barrage of short jokes with an endless supply of my favorite cartoons. From the comfort of my parents' bed, I blissfully emptied all my cares into bowls of cereal while Pinky and the Brain made another worthwhile and valiant attempt at taking over the world. I assumed that my dad wasn't paying attention to my favorite cartoon, but his next two questions proved he was indeed listening.

He started the conversation by asking, "Son, between Pinky and Brain, which one is the leader?"

This simple question made me think I had to inform him about the underlying premise of the show. In detail, I explained that Brain was certainly the leader and Pinky was more like the sidekick, the assistant, the gofer. Brain was clearly the leader, Brain was indispensable, Brain was "the brain" behind the whole operation. I gave my dad multiple examples to prove my point.

Now I realize I wasn't teaching him anything. Instead, he was shaping the next twenty years of my life while I ate cereal on a Saturday morning.

"OK," he said. "Between Pinky and Brain, which one is shorter?"

I responded with one word: "Brain."

My father ended the lesson by stating, "Always remember this, son: The short one is the leader. Pinky is tall, but Pinky is stupid. Those kids at school probably make fun of your height because they're jealous of your grades. One day you'll hire them to work for you."

If he'd had a mic, he could have dropped it.

Years later my dad took me to my first concert at the illustrious Boston Garden, surprising me with tickets to see a Kirk Franklin event. (At that point, only sixteen championship banners hung from the rafters.) As the concert began and the aroma of street foods like sausage, onions, and peppers filled the venue, I was completely engrossed and experienced slight sensory overload.

Then during intermission, my father asked me a question eerily reminiscent of an earlier life lesson. With a voice filled with curiosity, he asked, "Who's the leader on that stage?"

"Kirk Franklin," I answered. That was obvious. Although Kirk didn't sing, it was clear that he controlled everyone else's actions, like an orchestra conductor. The symphony of voices and instruments performed to Kirk's exact specifications. From time to time he would let random members of his choir sing the lead part, but their talents only seemed to make Kirk look more in control of the experience than ever. The dancing. The music. The singers. The band. They were all led by Kirk Franklin, so it was clear who the leader was.

My dad's next question revealed his intentions behind asking the first question. "Who's the shortest person on stage?"

"Kirk," I answered.

My father used this twofold line of reasoning throughout my formative years, and it worked. Throughout my childhood and into my teenage years, I equated shortness with leadership capacity because my dad brain washed me to think that way. The intimacy I had with my father gave him an open door to insert his ideas into my mind's operating system. Could it be that our minds are susceptible to viruses because there's no firewall protecting our intimate spaces from the influence of outside forces?

I was indeed short and always had been short. But my awareness of that alerted my father that my gaze was turning inward and he was no longer the only source of truth in my journey of self-discovery. How he rebounded from this deviation in my journey allowed him to steer the formation of my identity for years to come and still leaves me grateful to this day. He would have never had the ability to help form and guide my identity if he weren't within earshot. My dad's ideas were able to permeate my thinking because we were *just talking*.

We've examined the three levels of descent Adam falls into, and now we begin to climb out of independence, insecurity, and isolation by very closely examining the life of Jesus and the Mind of Christ. The Mind of Christ reveals a three-rung ladder to retrieve us from the cavern of Adam's darkness. The first rung is intimacy, the second is identity, and the final is interdependence.

I would have never been able to receive my dad's lessons regarding insecurities and the power of identity if we had lacked an intimate relationship. Intimacy was a nonnegotiable for identity formation and the renewal of my mind.

At times, it may feel as though we're skipping ahead to talk about identity, but we'll only preemptively glance forward in order to reveal how intimacy is oftentimes the overlooked and underestimated first step that propels us toward our identity. The identity-shaping conversations I had with my father were possible only because of our intimate relationship.

Friendship with God

Intimacy with God is the undeniable catalyst for adopting the Mind of Christ. It isn't necessarily easy or simple, but the good news is that it's attainable and worth all the obstacles we must overcome.

Our God has a long history of establishing intimate relationships with humanity. The short of it is that God is really into humans. Not only did He create us, which means He's intimately acquainted with our design, but He created us for relationship with Him and others.

Have you ever wondered why God rested on the seventh day? In Psalm 121 the Bible teaches that our God neither sleeps nor slumbers. He requires no rest, so He wouldn't have rested on the seventh day because of fatigue. What, then, had the power to make the Creator stop in His tracks? What could have possibly interrupted His schedule? What was so beautiful and captivating that God didn't continue with His work on the seventh day?

The sixth day marked the creation of humanity, and the seventh day was God's version of paternity leave. He took one look at the crown of His creation and immediately decided the next day would be dedicated to establishing intimacy between Himself and His humans. Like a child unwrapping gifts on Christmas morning, God was eager to interact with humanity, and so He declared that the seventh day would be a Sabbath. He was so enthralled with Adam and Eve that He rested so He could enjoy life with the humans He had created.

The Bible teaches us that God enjoys making friends and has given us a road map for establishing intimacy with Him. He considered Abraham His friend and was appalled by the thought of keeping secrets from him. Genesis 18:17 records that God said, "Shall I hide from Abraham what I am about to do?" There is no clearer sign of friendship and intimacy than the inability to keep a secret from someone! God also called Moses His friend. Exodus 33:11 reports, "The LORD would speak to Moses face to face, as one speaks to a friend."

God desires intimacy with His creation. He has a lot to say, and He wants to spread His ideas about life to us and personally rewire the way we think. But that can't happen outside of an intimate friendship with Him.

In order to adopt the Mind of Christ, we have to first adopt the habits of Christ and use His life as a blueprint for the pattern and pace of our lives. Jesus undeniably prioritized intimacy with God. Luke recorded that He "often withdrew to lonely places and prayed" (Luke 5:16). It's no surprise, then, that the ideas and thoughts of God came pouring from the mouth of Christ. Jesus was pregnant with wisdom, clarity, faith, and instruction because He was consistently intimate with God.

This level of friendship and intimacy isn't reserved just for Moses, Abraham, and Jesus. These accounts should encourage and inspire all of us because God rewards those who earnestly and diligently seek Him. Therefore, let's explore the three necessary ingredients for intimacy: time, talking, and trust.

When we spend time in the presence of God, enjoy conversations with God, and trust Him to the point of unconditional surrender and unwavering obedience, we are walking in intimacy. The ingredients of time, talking, and trust have the power to build intimacy and revolutionize the way we think. That's because whoever we're intimate with will inevitably impregnate us with their ideas.

Each ingredient is necessary to have true biblical intimacy. You may currently have two of the three ingredients nailed down, but it's the strong combination of this three-strand cord that won't be easily broken. Trust, talking, and time are the three nonnegotiables that form the bond of intimacy with God.

You may spend time with God and talk to Him, but if you don't trust Him enough to surrender your life to Him and obey Him, then you're not intimate.

You may trust God and enjoy talking to Him, but the daily discipline and consistency of spending time with Him is how you maintain, not just obtain, mental clarity. The Word of God is described in the Bible as food, and eating must be daily to be effective.

You may trust God and spend time with Him, but love longs to communicate. God certainly has the ability to read your mind, but He wants to hear your voice and wants your ear to be attuned to hearing His. Good conversations are never one-sided, and mind reading doesn't require any intimacy and doesn't build intimacy. Yes, God can easily read our minds, but He'd much rather change them, and that can happen only through intimate conversation.

Time

The first hurdle to overcome if we're going to build an intimate and close relationship with God is the investment of time. Intimacy is never convenient, requires a lot of time, and takes time. Intimacy doesn't happen quickly, nor will it flourish with inconsistent investments of time. Mark recorded that "very early in the morning, while it was still dark, Jesus got up, left the house and went off to a solitary place, where he prayed" (Mark 1:35). Jesus wanted uninterrupted quality time with God, so He woke up and left before anyone could request a miracle or ask a question.

We currently live in a microwavable culture, but intimacy with God can be formed only at Crock-Pot speeds. So often we bring our twenty-first-century technology and immediate expectations into a rather slow-paced, consistent relationship with God. Whiplash is common when people encounter God, because the pace is so different from what they're accustomed to. Simply put, God is not in a rush, but so often we are. Nothing with God happens quickly, and many people fade into the category of extended family, spending time with God only on holidays and special occasions. Every conversation is consumed with the goal of "catching up."

Talking

Second, intimacy demands conversation laced with transparency, openness, and honesty. King David is the poster child for transparent conversations with God. His prayers are littered throughout the book of Psalms, and they're raw and shockingly uncensored and unrehearsed. He admits his feelings of anger and rage. He confesses his doubts and fears. He's transparent when it comes to his desire for revenge. He bares his soul to God in a way that organized religion can't teach. Passages in 1 and 2 Samuel and 1 Chronicles reveal that David consistently "inquired of the Lord" to ask for wisdom and guidance when making key decisions.

Communication is a two-way street, and nothing is more frustrating than a one-sided conversation. God is love, and love longs to communicate. Intimacy with Him is developed when we talk to Him and then listen for His words for us. God speaks through His written Word so that we can become familiar with His spoken word.

Two distinct words in the original language of the Bible both mean "word": *logos* and *rhema*. Logos is the written Word of God. Rhema is the spoken word of God.

Communicating with God requires both logos and rhema, and they never contradict but always complement and complete each other. Jesus was incredible at hearing the rhema of God as well as recalling the logos of God, and both are necessary for an intimate relationship with God.

Trust

Last, trust is ultimately expressed in our ability to obey what God is asking of us. When Jesus tells His disciples they will keep His commands if they love Him (John 14:15), He makes it clear that love isn't simply a feeling. Unfortunately, our culture has made love about feelings—about stomach butterflies and physical attraction. Jesus, though, makes love about obedience, because obedience is the ultimate sign of trust. Obedience is the proof that we've relinquished our independence. Obedience is unconditional surrender.

I've learned that whenever there's disobedience, there's also distrust. The only reason we willingly, knowingly, and continually disobey God is that we trust ourselves more than we trust Him. Disobedience is the natural by-product of distrust, and it destroys intimacy between God and humans.

Jesus had the authority to teach this principle because He modeled it. Hours before His arrest, the reality of the crucifixion began to set in, and He wandered out to a nearby garden to pray. He would have inevitably witnessed a crucifixion or two during His lifetime, but now the weight and pressure of His own prolonged torture was imminent. To say that Jesus was stressed would be a gross understatement. The thought of being stripped and brutally broken apart crippled Him as blood formed on and dripped from His forehead.

Jesus must have lost control of His body as panic and fear overshadowed him.

Shaking hands.

Cold sweats.

Crippling fear.

Involuntary reactions.

Everything in Him wanted to run away. Human instinct wanted to bail on the predetermined plan. All strength evaporated.

As we've seen, gardens can attract snakes, and so the weakened state of our superhero created a perfect scenario for the Serpent to rack up another win. It should have been easy for him to push Jesus over the edge with this simple idea: *What father kills His son?* Then followed with *There must be another way,* laying out a clear path to independence and self-preservation.

When we operate under the Mind of Adam, we argue with God:

- We fight His will.
- We assert our will.
- We debate.
- We kick and scream.
- We rationalize.

But Jesus rejected the fruit:

- He rejected the Serpent's idea.
- He rejected the path to moral independence.
- He rejected His own opinion and modeled a path back to the Tree of Life for all of humanity.

Jesus demonstrated what life looks like when we're sober and no longer under the influence of the fruit Eve shared with Adam. This is the fruit of good theology. When we're absolutely certain that God is good, loving, perfect, and kind, we no longer have to find our own provision of fruit. We trust that God's monopoly on ideas is for our good, and we abandon the black market of half-truths and ideological concepts the Serpent has for sale next to the withered tree.

It's fitting that Jesus takes an axe to the root of the Tree of Knowledge in the garden of Gethsemane, because everything went haywire in a garden. He leads the rebellion against independence with radical trust in the character and will of God. He's tempted to save Himself, but His response to this temptation is beautiful: "Father, if you are willing, take this cup from me; yet not my will, but yours be done" (Luke 22:42).

Jesus submits Himself to be tortured.

Jesus submits Himself to be wrongfully imprisoned.

Jesus submits Himself to be hammered.

Jesus submits Himself to be crushed.

Jesus submits Himself to a long, slow death.

Why? Because it was the will of God, and He knew God was trustworthy. Jesus was "brain washed," and to be brain washed means you trust every word spoken by a leader—like hundreds of people trusted cult leader Jim Jones in the 1970s and gladly drank the "Kool-Aid." Jesus trusts His leader, the Father, so much that He's willing to accept death on a Roman cross and receive the penalty for humanity's sin.

Can you imagine this level of commitment?

Can you imagine surrendering your will in this way?

Can you imagine this kind of radical trust?

Like a toddler jumping off the kitchen counter into the arms of a loving parent, Jesus free falls into the arms of God and completely trusts that the will of the Father is a safe place. Jesus trusts His Father more than He trusts Himself.

Trust isn't a goal we achieve but rather the fruit we grow. Trust is the fruit that grows in the fertile soil of sustained intimacy with God. If intimacy is the soil, then our ideas are the seeds we sow in the garden of our minds.

The Mind of Christ submits the will of Christ to the divine will of the Father. The Mind of Christ is marked by trust, and recapturing the power of your mind begins with trusting the Father more than you trust yourself.

Jesus did not develop this kind of radical trust in a moment. There was a track record of trust and a journey of intimacy. The Mind of Christ can't be adopted without the lifestyle of Jesus. Our Savior and Lord developed rhythms in His life that allowed margin for spending intimate time with God. I've come to firmly believe that who you spend time with determines the ideas you entertain, and it's clear that throughout Jesus's life, His wisdom, understanding, and governing mindset reflected His sustained intimacy with the Father.

I have personally struggled a great deal with all three ingredients for intimacy, but of the three, trust has been the most difficult. So many circumstances have made me question whether God can even be trusted. I've had moments of great disappointment, such as times in hospitals when doctors delivered bad news and the crushing weight of despair was debilitating. But after walking with God for decades, I've realized that only immature Christians wonder whether He can be trusted.

The question isn't whether we can trust God; He's not a variable but a constant. The real question is whether God can trust us. We vary. We vacillate. We're unfaithful. We're inconsistent. The mature Christian is wondering whether God trusts him or her, not the other way around.

God can be trusted.

Humans, not so much.

Intimacy with God is the result of proving that we indeed trust Him and can be trusted by Him. The quicker we overcome the hurdle of trusting Him, the quicker we can start working on being trusted by Him.

I have had the privilege of making friends with a handful of people who happen to be incredibly wealthy, and I've learned a lot about them. First, they're insanely generous. Second, it takes them a long time to trust people.

I've realized the same two truths can be said concerning our God. First, He is insanely generous with His love, grace, mercy, and kindness. He sustains human life on this planet even for those who don't love or acknowledge Him.

Second, it takes a lot to gain God's trust. I've often mistaken the generosity of my wealthy friends for their trust. But they don't have to trust in order to act generously, and the same miscalculation can be made when observing God's generosity. God is generous because that's simply His nature. He's a giver, and just because He has blessed you with things doesn't mean He trusts you with His secrets like He trusted Abraham with them.

Now, if you're wondering whether God trusts you with His secrets, you should simply consider whether you've ever found yourself on top of a mountain with what you love most strapped to an altar to test your allegiance. Abraham was willing to sacrifice Isaac because he trusted God, and in return God started trusting Abraham, which created the kind of intimacy that always impregnates us with God-ideas.

Intimacy is certainly intimidating.

Intimacy is also inconvenient.

But intimacy impregnates our barren minds. It ultimately leads to ideas' indoctrination. It produces imitation.

Lastly, intimacy prepares us for identity.

Brain Washed

Cult leaders like Jim Jones aren't the only maniacal villains who exploit others by brain washing them. Dictators are notorious for brain washing their citizens. From Kim Jong-un of North Korea to Adolf Hitler in Nazi Germany, dictators are known for weaponizing information, utilizing propaganda, and brain washing their people to believe in the leader's delusion of utopia. One could argue that to be a dictator one must develop and wield some advanced brainwashing skills or else totalitarian regimes would crumble quicker than a stale cookie.

The word *dictator* comes from the Latin word *dictatour*, which means "Roman chief magistrate with absolute authority." However, the root of the word is another Latin word, *dictare*, which means "to say often, prescribe."[1] By definition, then, a dictator is someone who controls with absolute authority by using their words. The root of *dictator* is simply *dictate*, and it is the gift of words that makes brain washing possible. All dictators have set themselves up to be gods and therefore idols. They all attempt to do what only our God can rightfully accomplish.

Genesis tells us that our God spoke creation into existence with His word. He formed and organized the solar system with His word. His word doesn't return to Him empty but accomplishes every task for which it is sent (Isaiah 55:11). So this God sent His word to His creation, and "the Word became flesh and made his dwelling among us" (John 1:14). Jesus is amazed at the centurion because the man believes in the power of Jesus's spoken word (Matthew 8:10). Of course, this Word-Became-Flesh-God-Man would instruct His disciples to ensure that He—and His words—remained in them (John 15:4–5). We'll talk more about that later.

> Our God has the power to renew our minds because He dictates.
> Our God rules over the cosmos through dictation.
> Our God brain washes His sons and daughters through dictation.

The word *dictator* has negative connotation because no human being has the character to hold absolute power without becoming absolutely corrupt. Our God, however, is no mortal. He's a loving Father with absolute authority, and your next step toward mental freedom is found in the words of our God. His logos. His rhema. Whether His dictated words achieve their intended outcome will be determined by your distance. So get close and let Him dictate your identity and future.

PART TWO

Adopting the Mind of Christ

5

The Maker's Mark

Yet to all who did receive him, to those who believed in his name, he gave the right to become children of God.

John 1:12

Then God said, "Let us make mankind in our image, in our likeness, so that they may rule."

Genesis 1:26

God made him who had no sin to be sin for us, so that in him we might become the righteousness of God.

2 Corinthians 5:21

The glory of God is man fully alive.

Irenaeus

IMAGINE STANDING AT THE ENTRANCE to a dark room, dumbfounded at the odd scene of someone grabbing, grasping, and grappling with the darkness, trying to force it into trash bins. You enter the room and ask them to explain what they're doing.

"Isn't it obvious?" they reply. "I'm trying to get rid of all the darkness in here."

After the initial shock, you alert them of an easier way to get rid of the darkness. You walk over to a switch and simply turn on the lights. The person is completely blown away, so you explain that darkness isn't a material substance but rather the absence of light. Darkness can't be gathered, collected, or handled because it exists only in the void of light.

The scene I just described may seem idiotic and senseless, yet I've encountered hundreds if not thousands of people who approach their insecurities in the exact same manner. They focus all their attention on "getting rid of" them. But insecure thoughts, like darkness, are the result of an absence, and they aren't as substantive as you may think.

Insecure thoughts can form only in the void created by a lack of identity. Identity, like light, has the power to dispel and destroy insecure thoughts. Therefore, this chapter will focus on practical steps for receiving your true identity from the only source that could provide it—your Creator. Your insecurities are no more intimidating than the darkness, and this chapter will place the light switch of God's truth concerning your identity within your grasp.

The genesis of true confidence and identity can never begin with the examination of creation but must start with thoughts about the Creator. Humans were created in the image of God, and we are by nature a reflection of Him. Therefore, any rejection of Him completely destroys our chances of accepting ourselves because a rejection of the image will inevitably result in a rejection of the reflection.

But once we conclude that our Creator is good, perfect, wise, and loving, it becomes effortless to conclude that anything made by Him must be up to par with His standards. The foundation of our identity as created beings is found in the fundamental truth that God cannot create anything that isn't good. That's because *He* is good, and His indelible fingerprint is found on everything He's created. Our sense of value doesn't come from within ourselves; it's been eternally set by the One who has created and redeemed us. Everything created by Him bears the Maker's mark and has infinite intrinsic value.

Ultimately, when we spend intimate time with God, we desire to be more like Him. We discern His image within us, and it drives us to become more like Him. Intimacy with God causes us to identify with Him. In the context of intimacy, we realize that although God is divinely different from us, He has created us in His likeness, and that knowing and valuing Him is the key for knowing and valuing ourselves. Until we identify with Him through intimate relationship, we will always reject identity from Him.

On this leg of the journey, we will receive and recover our God-given identity, and our insecurities will fade into nothing.

So Who Are We?

Three crucial pillars of truth bear the weight of our God-given identity, and we must accept all three to fully adopt the Mind of Christ.

First, we must believe and accept that we are children of God. While Jesus walked through the streets of Jerusalem and the countryside of Judea, He walked in the confidence of sonship, and we must follow suit.

Second, we must understand the power of the image of God living within us. When God created Adam and Eve, His image was woven into the fabric of their souls and central to their original design.

Last, based on the sacrificial death of Jesus, we have become the righteousness of God.

We are the children of God, we are made in the image of God, and we are the righteousness of God. The by-product of identifying with our God is that we can rest from the pursuit of trying to discover who we are. You may notice that all three identifications for humanity include how we specifically relate to God. Indeed, humans only have identity as beings that are in relation to the Creator. We are His children, made in His image, displaying His righteousness. Our identity is found only in our connection to Him.

Confidence in Its Rightful Place

As the youth pastor, nothing made me more nervous than having to confront and discipline one of my pastor's triplet boys. (That's right, triplet boys, all of whom were actively involved in our youth ministry.)

One Wednesday night our volunteers alerted me that one of the triplets—who shall remain nameless for purposes of this illustration—had just been taking snacks from our "bodega" without paying for them. I could barely be angry with them for not stopping the kid because I didn't even want to stop him. But he and I had a two-minute conversation that marked me for years.

I walked up to him and said, "Hey, man, I heard you took some snacks from the bodega without paying for them."

He responded, "Yup."

I really didn't know where to go from there. I had never had a student admit to anything so quickly. After a short pause, I said, "Well, you gotta start bringing money if you want stuff from the bodega."

Without pausing, his knee-jerk reaction was, "My dad owns the bodega."

I should have gone to our media booth for a mic and handed it to him just so he could drop it. The kid reminded me of what I already knew—his status as a son. He didn't tell me anything about himself; he just reminded me of who his father was—even if he was wrong about his dad actually owning the bodega.

Although I was impressed, I wasn't willing to lose ground. So I told him, "If your dad *owns* the bodega, then he's probably wealthy enough to give you money for snacks, right?"

He returned what he'd taken, and the next week he was prepared to buy as many snacks as his cavities would allow. I returned the next week with a deeper understanding of what it looks like to walk in the mental authority of sonship.

Although I didn't agree with this kid's actions, I did admire his confidence. He believed and claimed that he had a right to take snacks without paying for them because of his dad's position and status. He didn't justify his actions by telling me how creative he was. He didn't mention his grades from the previous semester. And he could've tried to impress me by telling me the snacks were for his new girlfriend or used his charisma and charm, but he didn't.

None of that held any weight in his mind, because he believed his relationship to his father made the difference. He placed no confidence in himself or his accomplishments but had complete confidence in his dad's authority. I was forced to correct his activity, but I was in awe of his mentality.

I wish we were all a little bit more like him. My fear is that most times when we teach on confidence, we're calling people to place confidence in themselves instead of in who they are in relation to God. Identity is never formed in the vacuum of isolation from God but only in context of our relationship with Him.

This incident prompted me to ask what my Father owns. He owns "the cattle on a thousand hills" (Psalm 50:10). The Bible says, "The earth is the LORD's, and all its fullness" (Psalm 24:1 NKJV). And in Ezekiel 18:4 the Lord says, "Behold, all souls are mine," so every human being under the sun belongs to God.

Do you assume that God's authority is your inheritance? Jesus did. In the parable of the two sons, also known as the parable of the prodigal son, the father was clearly disappointed with the bitter and legalistic attitude of his older son. Yet he still asserted to him, "Everything I have is yours" (Luke 15:31).

Clearly, this pastor's son understood that everything belonging to his father was also his, even though he was a bit confused about the bodega.

This is the principle Peter used when he responded to a man begging for money: "Silver or gold I do not have, but what I do have I give you. In the name of Jesus Christ of Nazareth, walk" (Acts 3:6). Peter gave the man more than he asked for because he knew the power he possessed as a son of God. How many people in our broken world remain crippled because they don't believe the fullness of what they possess as coheirs with Christ?

The confidence I saw this young man walk in is the confidence that all sons and daughters walk in when they adopt the Mind of Christ. Could it be that every time I've doubted myself, I was actually doubting whether I was a legitimate son of God? Could it be that I've wasted time trying to believe in myself when all that's necessary to walk in confidence is to be certain of who my Father is?

The confidence to walk in the authority of our adoption flows directly from the intimacy we form with the Father, and our intimacy with God is most influenced by our ideas of God. In order to establish intimacy, we must neglect the inclination toward independence and approach God as dependent beings in need of a loving Father.

This kid reminded me of Jesus that night, because Jesus walked in the same kind of boldness and confidence that I find to be so evident throughout the Gospels.

We'll explore the confident sonship of Jesus more fully later.

The Maker's Mark

We interact with the power of branding every single day, and the world's most influential companies understand the importance of a great logo. The moment your eye catches the slightest glimpse of the green and white Starbucks siren, the double-tailed mermaid draws you in and magically causes you to crave lattes and pastries. The hidden white arrow created by the negative space between the *E* and *X* subliminally causes us to associate FedEx with speed and precision. When I was growing up, the absence of the Nike swoosh logo or the Timberland tree on sports or outdoors wear was non-negotiable means for a lunchroom roasting session. Whether or not we like it, logos and brand design matter, and the most powerful companies know this.

That explains why Disney has a team of lawyers who will hunt you down if you dare use their logo improperly or without their permission. The power of branding is evidenced by the $211,000,000 that BP, the oil and gas company, paid a group of creative ad and PR agencies to create a new logo for them.[1]

The ultimate goal of every brand is for their logo to become synonymous with their name, which explains why Starbucks removed its name from their logo in 2011. The siren finally had the power to stand on her "own two feet" without the name of the company surrounding the logo. When we see the golden arches, we immediately begin to crave perfectly salted french fries, no name necessary. And a red bull's-eye is all you need to see before your car is magnetically pulled into the parking lot of a one-stop-shop superstore.

The human brain processes pictures and images much faster than it can process words. Therefore, logos have the potential to immediately deliver positive- or negative-associated memories, emotions, and thoughts to your brain, and a decision to purchase is literally seconds away.

But none of these globally recognizable brands were the first to capitalize on the power of strategic marketing, branding, and logo creation. God beat them all to the punch. The book of Genesis informs us that "God said, 'Let us make mankind in our image, in our likeness, so that they may rule'" (Genesis 1:26).

Humans were created in the image and likeness of God to be His logo on the colony of Earth. The sight of a human being is supposed to immediately cause the viewer to think about God. In the same way that a successful logo no longer needs the accompanying name of the company it represents, humans were created to immediately point creation toward its Creator. You are a logo for the Divine. You are a poster child for heaven's kingdom and culture. To be human is to be endowed with the Maker's mark, which communicates our intrinsic value and worth. That is the truth concerning your identity, and the image of God imprinted on your soul means more than your race, gender, socioeconomic status, or any other grain of sand on which you've built your identity.

Again, Genesis 1:26 records that "God said, 'Let us make mankind in our image, in our likeness, so that they may rule.'" The only way to properly understand the true meaning of these words is to recover the original meaning to the original recipients of the Genesis account. What would they have thought about based on hearing the words *image* and *likeness*? What ideas would these words trigger in their minds?

The original audience of the Bible's account of creation, traditionally credited to Moses, would have been familiar with the terms *image* and *likeness* because God always communicates using common vernacular. Just because the meaning of a passage may not be immediately obvious to us doesn't mean the meaning was lost on the original recipients. We must remember that although the Bible was written *for* us, it was not originally written *to* us.

When the original audience heard the words *image* and *likeness*, they would have immediately thought of kings, empires, and taxes. In many ancient imperial scenarios, a king or emperor resided within the capital city of the empire while most of its inhabitants lived in distant cities and lands far away from the capital.

Let's take King Nebuchadnezzar, for instance. He resided within the glorious city of Babylon, yet the vast Babylonian Empire stretched from the Mediterranean all the way to the Persian Gulf. That meant most of the inhabitants of that empire would never personally lay eyes on their emperor.

Well, how were they supposed to believe in someone they never saw?

Simple solution. Statues would be constructed in the image and likeness of the emperor and then placed all over the empire. Citizens may never see the emperor, but they would indeed interact with his image. The statue was an instant reminder of in whose kingdom the citizens were in fact residing.

Coinage followed this same logic. Jesus lived within the Roman Empire, which was ruled by Caesar. Jesus and His disciples would have never seen Caesar in person, but they were keenly aware of his power because every single time they purchased something, they had to use coins that bore Caesar's image. The coin was made in the image of the one who controlled the currency.

So when God wanted to help His people understand their identity, He used language that would make the concept easy to grasp. They were familiar with empires, statues, and coins. They were familiar with "image" and "likeness" the same way we're familiar with logos and branding.

The capitol and center of God's kingdom is not Planet Earth. The kingdom of heaven revolves around the throne of God. But there is a way for the inhabitants of Earth to become aware of the King's power and presence. God created humans in His image and likeness so His will, culture, and power would be at work even in His absence.

God is King, and we are His regional governors, endowed with His authority as evidenced by the Maker's mark on our souls. Genesis tells us exactly why God created humans in His image and likeness and clearly states that it was for the sole purpose of ruling over this colony called Earth. The Serpent wasn't too thrilled about his subjugated status, so he found a way to rob Adam and Eve of their authority: He stained them with the crimson smear of sin. God designed us to be fashionable and functional. We were made in His image in order to rule in His place and in His likeness to reflect His beauty and glory.

The statue reminded every citizen of who was in charge.

The coins made everyone mindful of to whom they owed taxes.

When God made humans in His image, it was for the central purpose of colonizing Earth. However, the peripheral by-product is found in the exalted value placed on human life. Our worth and value aren't found in the dirt we come from but in the divine breath that caused us to come to life.

Unfortunately, we attempt to build our sense of self-worth on our dirt instead of taking inventory on our divine breath.

We all bear the Maker's mark. We've been branded and are walking logos for the Creator. That is our identity.

Once Nebuchadnezzar died or experienced defeat and was overthrown by a new ruler, the statues made in his image and likeness were rendered obsolete. Once Caesar ceased to be the emperor, the coins simply became collector's items. We have dethroned God, yet we wonder why we struggle to find meaning, value, and identity. Our identity is dependent on the One to whom we are eternally tethered, and placing God on the thrones of our hearts will also repair the brokenness of our self-valuation.

True Conviction

Every once in a while, my wife calls me Pastor Manny, which alerts me that I've done something unbecoming of my pastoral office.

When I make fun of someone.

When I completely lose my cool while driving.

When I say something blatantly unbiblical.

I am made keenly aware of my mistake when I hear Tia say, "Really, Pastor Manny?" Her tone communicates that she expects better from someone with my level of influence and spiritual maturity. But although she's confronting me, she's actually complimenting me. That's because nothing is more insulting than a lack of high expectations from someone. In those moments when my wife reminds me of my identity, she's convicting me of righteousness.

John 16:8 is a beautiful verse where Jesus teaches that "when [the Holy Spirit] has come, He will convict the world of sin, and of righteousness, and of judgment" (NKJV). The sobering part of the verse is that the Holy Spirit will convict the world of sin and judgment. No escaping that part. But that's not the only thing the Bible declares the Holy Spirit will convict us of. He will convict us of our righteousness, which is essentially what my wife does when she reminds me that I'm a pastor. The Holy Spirit will remind us that our sinful actions don't make much sense based on the righteous status we have with God.

I've discovered a beautiful truth about humans, and it's the lynchpin argument of this entire book: People only act in accordance with what they believe about themselves.

Simply put, belief before behavior.

The Bible understands this truth, which explains why Proverbs 23:7 reminds us that "as he thinks in his heart, so is he" (NKJV). Even industrialist Henry Ford understood this fact when he said, "Whether you think you can, or you think you can't—you're right."

Behavior doesn't produce belief. Rather, belief predicts behavior. Therefore, God cements our status as righteous, even before our actions can catch up, because He wants us to believe we are righteous. He understands that humans only act in accordance with what they believe about themselves. If we believe we are the righteousness of God, we will inevitably act righteous. Therefore, when John 16:8 declares that the Spirit of Truth (as named in verse 13) will convict us of righteousness, we shouldn't be surprised. God's conviction is never condemnation. His conviction is always a reminder of our true identity and a challenge to stop living beneath heaven's imperial standard.

Researchers have learned that teachers can affect a student's potential for achievement by treating them according to their expectations of that student. One study "found that expectations affect teachers' moment-to-moment interactions with the children they teach in a thousand almost invisible ways."[2] So if a teacher believes a student is capable of success, that student is more likely to succeed. But if a teacher believes a student is capable of only failure, that student is more likely to fail.

When we're treated like a success, then, we can believe in ourselves and rise to meet the level of expectation. Conversely, though, when we're treated like a failure, we can believe we're a failure and then fail.

God doesn't call us sinful.

God doesn't treat us like we're sinful.

God doesn't expect us to act sinful.

God calls us His righteousness.

Paul teaches the Corinthian church about their true identity when he writes that "God made him who had no sin to be sin for us, so that in him we might become the righteousness of God" (2 Corinthians 5:21). This final pillar must be in place so we can accurately identify ourselves based on the truth of God's verdict concerning our status. Whatever you believe about yourself is exactly what you'll become.

We are children of God.

We were made in the very image and likeness of God.

We are the righteousness of God.

We must be convinced of who we are.

These are the pillars of our identity. These should determine how you think about yourself.

Purpose Is Not Identity

I never realized how cold microphones can be until I picked one up to preach my first sermon in front of a live audience. My sweaty palms quickly melted the frigid metal microphone into an instrument of destiny that Thursday night right after my thirteenth birthday.

I can still remember everything about that evening. I had preached in the shower, in my room, and in front of my mirror, but this was the first time I felt my heart pounding within my frail teenage chest. Nobody told me how difficult it was to control your breathing when you're nervous. I was even nervous about sounding nervous, which inevitably made me sound nervous.

But soon after I started, the crowd warmed up. I got them to laugh, and then I fired off the few Bible verses I knew. I got really fired up like all the good preachers I had watched and got a standing ovation. With the microphone in one hand and a Bible in the other, I moved the room, and I've never stopped preaching.

I was born to preach, and I'm a natural leader with a loud voice. My first-grade teacher constantly used me to make classroom announcements and rally my class. I was also a regularly scheduled reader during DEAR time. (DEAR stands for the Drop Everything And Read program. Maybe it was just my school? *Kanye aka Ye shrug.*)

Not only was I a natural leader and loudmouth, but I read better than most of my classmates because my mother was slightly obsessed with teaching me.

I have two much older half-siblings from my mother's first marriage, but my parents wrestled with infertility for years and even suffered a miscarriage. With tears of joy cascading down her full brown cheeks, my mother explained to me that, after her miscarriage, she'd prayed, *God, if You give me a son, I'll give him back to You.*

The fact that she would even pray is mind-blowing because she wasn't yet a believer or born again. She even prayed a theologically accurate prayer!

When she did have a son—me—she tried her best to deliver on her end of the bargain she'd made with this invisible God she didn't even know. Through the years she taught me to read using the Bible, dropped me off at an African Methodist Episcopal Church, enrolled me in a Catholic school, and sent me to a Pentecostal youth group. From the time I was six until I graduated college with my bachelor's degree in theological and biblical studies, she reminded me weekly that I was destined to be a preacher, that God had placed me on this planet to preach, and that I was to be wholly dedicated to God for the sole purpose of preaching and teaching His Word.

My identity was completely built on the foundation that I was a preacher of God's Word. First and foremost, I saw myself as a preacher, and I assumed that since preaching was a noble task, obviously being a preacher would be a healthy identity to build my sense of self around. People proudly use so many negative identity markers, but I chose to build my life on a very positive one.

From the time I was thirteen onward, the one word I would have used to describe my identity, my passions, my gifts, and my destiny without blinking an eye would have been *preacher*. I preached on a regular basis, and by the time I was fifteen, I was good enough to preach at our church's annual Good Friday Youth Conference. Thousands of young people from across the city of Boston would pour into New Covenant Christian Church to hear the gospel preached, and I always ended up with the microphone, preaching there throughout the rest of my teenage years.

Then when I was twenty, a new youth pastor had arrived at the church, and as Good Friday approached, I realized that nobody had mentioned what my conference role or responsibilities would be.

So being the outspoken and assertive leader that I am, I pulled aside the youth pastor, who was twice my age, and made it known that I was ready to discuss my role for the youth conference. The youth pastor thanked me and assured me that I would be informed in a timely matter, and I began preparing content based on the theme of that year's conference.

The night before Good Friday, I figured I should attend the dress rehearsal. And to my shock, I learned that this new youth pastor had chosen other youth leaders to preach instead of me.

I felt deceived, betrayed, and broken. Preaching was my world. Preaching was my identity. I felt like I had just returned to the parking spot where I knew I'd left my car only to find an empty space. I felt robbed. I was angry, and I was tempted to boycott the event. To make matters worse, that same youth pastor refused to let me preach the entire duration of their tenure, and for two solid years of my life, I felt like Zechariah, whom the angel Gabriel pronounced mute.

At the time, I hated being silenced, muted, disregarded, and feeling like I had been thrown away and tossed aside. I felt like one of Andy's old toys from the movie *Toy Story*, alone in the attic, rejected and replaced. I felt like I had nothing to live for, I was depressed and broken, and my decisions started to reflect that. I began making unwise decisions regarding my relationships.

In the middle of that season, God pierced through the empty darkness and revealed His Father heart toward me. The voice of our heavenly Father is always unmistakable because it sounds so contrary to what we've been telling ourselves. God's message was so simple, so profound, and so radically different from what I had believed up until that point. He told me that if I never preached again, He'd still love me because I wasn't primarily a preacher but His son. He began to reveal and explain that my identity could not be found in preaching but only as His child.

So often we're busy, ambitiously building our Babel towers under the assumption that God is pleased. Many of us attempt to build our lives and our identities on our careers, our spouses, our wealth, or our gifts. Others of us never build anything because we're focused on our past, our sin, our failures, and our imperfections.

But regardless of in which one of the aforementioned groups you find yourself, God has the same solution. Your life and identity can never be built on self, whether on positive attributes of self or on negative attributes of self.

My entire solar system was orbiting around my ability to exegete Scripture, move a crowd, and deliver a good sermon. My identity was based on how well I performed, and I had to learn that performance-based validation is dysfunctional and unhealthy. Moreover, it's prohibited because Paul clearly tells us to place "no confidence in the flesh" (Philippians 3:3). Preaching was indeed my purpose. But I learned that purpose and identity are not synonymous or interchangeable terms the hard way. I had fallen into the common trap of using my purpose as my identity.

Whenever we're unaware of our true identity as sons and daughters of God, we grab the next best thing, which is our purpose. I know so many people who have built their entire lives around their career, calling, vocation, and purpose. I know pastors who have dedicated their whole lives to their calling but lost their families because they built their identity on the sinking sand of their purpose.

Looking back, I can now identify my actions and my emotional immaturity as insecure. I learned in that season that even God's call on our lives can become an idol, keeping us from experiencing true identity, which is found only in Christ. The objects of our idolatry aren't always inherently evil; there's nothing wrong with humans simply enjoying what God has provided. But idolatry begins when our hands start to close around an inherently good blessing from our God, arousing His jealousy.

Let's recall the story of Abraham being told to sacrifice his son Isaac. Isaac was a blessing from God, but Abraham was told to make him a burnt offering to prove that Isaac had not become an idol. Abraham and Sarah were permitted to enjoy their son as a blessing from God, but Isaac could not become the sole object of their souls' affections. God takes pleasure in His people enjoying His creation, but once we begin to worship and adore created things, we're dangerously close to building the foundation of our identity on the sinking sand of an idol instead of the cornerstone of Jesus Christ.

In my personal journey, I had to realize that the gift to preach and preaching itself were created things that had the power to exalt the Creator, but equally had the power to become idols in my life.

Confidence Amid Temptation

Immediately after Jesus's baptism, the Serpent appears to tempt Him. The same Serpent that deceived Adam and Eve into eating the forbidden fruit comes to tempt Jesus to eat bread, but the temptation has nothing to do with hunger and everything to do with intimacy and identity.

The Serpent finds Jesus in the wilderness and takes advantage of the opportunity. Matthew 4:3 tells us, "The tempter came to him and said, 'If you are the Son of God, tell these stones to become bread.'"

Do you see what the Serpent is doing? He's setting the same trap that worked against Adam and Eve. A cloud of paternal mystery had remained over Jesus's head until people heard the audible voice of God break into time and space at His baptism and call Him "my Son" (Matthew 17:5). But ignoring that confirmation, the Serpent decided to try to sow doubt.

The temptation isn't about food.

The temptation is about belief.

Just like in the garden.

The Serpent says, "If you are the Son of God, tell these stones to become bread." Can you hear the deception and manipulation in this question?

The Serpent attacks the most sensitive area in Jesus's life. He's saying, "If you are the Son of God, prove it."

But by trying to prove it, Jesus would have only shown that He didn't believe the truth God had declared at His baptism. He would've proven that His feelings or opinion held more weight than God's word.

But confidence is always silent.

Confidence feels no pressure to prove anything.

Jesus triumphed over the Serpent because He was confident in God's rhema. His brain had been washed.

Logos and Rhema

Jesus's response to the Serpent must be our model for establishing mental mastery. He said, "It is written: 'Man shall not live on bread alone, but on every word that comes from the mouth of God'" (Matthew 4:4). Jesus first responds by saying, "It is written," which is a clear reference to the written Word of God that Jesus used to establish intimacy with God. Next, Jesus declares that bread wouldn't suffice to meet His needs anyway, because humanity was designed to live and be nourished by the words that proceed from the mouth of God, a reference to the spoken word of God.

As I outlined earlier, *logos* is the written Word of God, and *rhema* is the spoken word of God. And logos and rhema make up the double-barreled weapon against the Serpent's thoughts and ideas. Reading the words of God. Hearing the words of God. Both work in tandem to renew our minds and protect our minds.

Do you struggle with insecure thoughts?

Are you plagued by depressing thoughts?

Are you constantly dealing with thoughts of comparison?

Do you battle against doubtful or fear-filled thoughts?

If so, you need more logos and more rhema. They work in tandem.

They're God's chosen modes of influence for us to adopt His thoughts.

The book of Isaiah is very clear on this:

> "For my thoughts are not your thoughts,
>   neither are your ways my ways,"
>   declares the LORD.
> "As the heavens are higher than the earth,
>   so are my ways higher than your ways
>   and my thoughts than your thoughts." (Isaiah 55:8–9)

When we expose ourselves to the logos and rhema of God on a daily basis, He begins to elevate our thinking. God wants to be the greatest influence over our thoughts, and He alone deserves that role in our lives because His thoughts transcend ours. Allowing God to influence the way we think is the surest way to stop the Serpent from infiltrating our minds and driving us toward doubt, rebellion, and independence. I believe this is why Jesus "often withdrew to lonely places and prayed" (Luke 5:16).

Jesus established a relational rhythm in His life that gave Him consistent access to God's rhema and logos. If He needed to withdraw to be with God often, why do we assume we can get by with less of God? Are we stronger than Jesus? I think not. Dependence on the Father's influence requires humility. If we believe we can figure things out on our own, we won't put in the work to receive from God. Jesus was keenly aware that without God's influence, the human mind would be easily manipulated by the Serpent.

This is why Jesus's advice to His disciples includes a command to remain in a state of dependence. In John 15:5–7 He declares, "I am the vine; you are the branches. If you remain in me and I in you, you will bear much fruit; apart from me you can do nothing. . . . If you remain in me and my words remain in you, ask whatever you wish, and it will be done for you."

Whereas Adam chose independence, those who are brain washed by God continually choose to remain dependent on His Word as the source of life. The words of God have become the Tree of Life for those who believe.

In these verses, Jesus makes it clear that intimacy with God is a prerequisite for any kind of mental success. He blatantly alerts His disciples that "apart from me you can do nothing," and then the passage takes an interesting turn based on how God decides to dwell within the life of the disciples. Jesus says that His words must remain in them. His rhema. His logos. Words are the fruit that grows from the soil of intimacy, and within the fruit of each word we find the new seeds necessary to secure our minds against the Serpent's agenda.

In Romans 12:2, the apostle Paul teaches that we are transformed by the renewing of our minds, and I've discovered that renewal can't occur separate from an intimate, influential, and dependent relationship with God.

Renewal requires relationship.

God had "brain washed" Jesus into confidently believing His position as the Son, the foundation of His entire identity. He performed miracles from the position of sonship, preached in the authority derived from sonship, and was consistently telling His disciples that they, too, were sons of God. Sonship is the cerebral cortex of the Mind of Christ.

Jesus's assertion of His identity was radical—and miraculous—considering the backdrop of His unique family dynamics. Earlier I mentioned the cloud of paternal controversy that had hung over His head for much of His life. Many of His contemporaries sarcastically referred to Him as "the carpenter's son" since Joseph was His stepfather (Matthew 13:55). Similar familial controversy would leave most people with a gaping emptiness in their soul and foundational cracks in their identity. But Jesus overcame every obstacle that life without an earthly father could have presented and stood firm in

His true identity as the Son of God. He invites all of humanity to do the same. The Mind of Christ is full of identity because Jesus overcame all forms of insecurity.

Jesus had no doubt heard the jokes about Mary's "fabricated fable and delusions of purity" and eavesdropped while His siblings mockingly called Him their half-brother. Jesus overheard the town gossip about His mom's mysterious "baby daddy" who had robbed Joseph of having a pure bride on their wedding night. Jesus had every reason to be insecure, yet every account we receive portrays a man who was "brain washed" concerning His identity as a Son and His relation to the heavenly Father. The weapon of insecurity was formed, but it certainly didn't prosper.

When it comes to the topics of identity formation, insecurity, and fatherhood, we would be wise to "let this mind be in [us] which was also in Christ Jesus" (Philippians 2:5 NKJV). The Mind of Christ on display for us in the Gospels is a mind that rejects insecurities, is brain washed concerning sonship and spiritual adoption, and longs for intimacy as well as identity from God the Father. The Mind of Christ found in Jesus is in clear juxtaposition with the Mind of Adam found in the parable of the two sons.

I'm convinced that no title or identity marker was closer to the bedrock of Jesus's self-evaluation of His identity than the royal and regal title of Son. The Mind of Christ orbits around the identity of sonship and is anchored by that identity. But the Mind of Adam seeks the same elusive goal as the people of Babel when they began to build a tower to reach the heavens so they could "make a name" for themselves (Genesis 11:4). Jesus felt no such pressure to build a tower or a name for Himself but rested in the power of His position as the Son.

King

Messiah

Prince of Peace

Savior

Healer

Anointed One

Emmanuel

Rabbi

Jesus was called by many titles, and all those titles are true and accurate. Yet when God decided to rend the heavens at Jesus's baptism, only one title was given—that of Son. Jesus identified Himself as the resurrection and the life, the way, the truth, the light of the world, and the true vine. But the title that provides a firm foundation for the others to rest on is the simple title of Son.

Could it be that the title we esteem the least is the name Jesus held closest to His heart? Is it possible that the parable of the two sons is really an invitation into true identity, found only as a child of God? Could it be that like the two sons, we want to be known as more than *just* sons and daughters of God? Could it be that all the title grabbing, name dropping, compliment fishing, and social-ladder climbing is a result of our refusal to accept the one piece of identity that everything else is built on?

The Mind of Christ was formed in the humanity of Jesus in a distinct order. The process of emotional and mental maturity we find modeled in the person of Jesus Christ is threefold. First and foremost, we find that Jesus established an intimate relationship with the Father. He established a rhythm to His life as a human that centers around spiritual disciplines and intentional intimacy with the Father. Whether those disciplines were consistent prayer times or in-depth Torah study, it's clear that by the age of twelve He had spent so much time with the Father that "everyone who heard him was amazed at his understanding and his answers" (Luke 2:47). Even at that young age, Jesus had an intimate relationship with the Father, which inevitably led to this confident twelve-year-old telling His biological parents who His real Father was.

Intimacy leads to the next phase of emotional and mental maturity, which is identity formation. Intimacy with the Father causes children of God to identify with God and receive identity from Him. Only intimacy causes us to truly desire God and to be like Him. Intimacy always produces identity within us, because only when we behold the glory of the Father are we truly proud and content with being His children.

Jesus was securely established in the approval of His Father.

Before any miracles were performed, He was approved of and accepted by God as His Son.

Before any crowds were preached to, He was approved of and accepted by God as His Son.

Before the triumphal entry, or Gethsemane, or Calvary, He was approved of and accepted by God as His Son.

Jesus walked in the security of divine approval and the identity of sonship.

So many of us settle for an insecure, pride-ridden, arrogant life, which really isn't life at all. The Mind of Christ offers divine approval, which leads to identity, humility, confidence, and true abundant life.

The Mind of Christ is full of approval, and it operates on the fuel of approval. But the Mind of Adam operates on the fuel of applause. Guilt, shame, and doubt fill the Mind of Adam, causing us to lust after the applause of others.

The journey from the Mind of Adam to the Mind of Christ starts with moving from the applause of men to the approval of God. I've found that once a person really believes and accepts the approval of God, their aching need for applause shrivels and dies.

Nicodemus and Jesus

Nicodemus, the religious leader we meet in John 3, was not as fortunate as Jesus was when it came to the formation of a biblically accurate identity. Jesus had the ability to preach with unparalleled power and conviction to thousands at a time, but He also had the love and compassion to meet people right where they happened to be and transform their perspective through dialogue and discussion.

Jesus never lost sight of the importance of each individual. Even in the midst of captivating large crowds, those crowds never seemed to captivate Christ. Whether He was going out of His way to talk with a Samaritan woman at a well or promising paradise to the thief hanging next to Him during the crucifixion, His conversations packed as much of a punch as His sermons.

One night Jesus makes time to talk to Nicodemus, and one of Jesus's comments has become so famous that apparel chain Forever 21 places the verse on the bottom of their shopping bags.

It's slightly controversial that Nicodemus is even interested in speaking with Jesus. Nicodemus identifies himself as a Pharisee, representing a group comprising Jesus's biggest opponents. Nicodemus's colleagues are critics, tireless in their verbal attacks of Jesus throughout the Gospels. The Pharisees are outspoken against His ministry, critical of the company He keeps, and doubtful concerning His claims of divine sonship, all while actively protesting His message in order to turn the hearts of people away from the Messiah.

Nicodemus, however, is curious. And though his contemporaries are doubtful, he can't deny the validity of Jesus's claims. He's caught in the crosshairs of the most pivotal and consequential religious debate in human history.

So Nicodemus carves out space and time to secretly meet with Jesus under the cover of night. He wouldn't dare meet with Him during the light of day; that would spark an uproar among his religious cronies and place his social status in jeopardy. He's not willing to neglect all the social clout he's built up over the years for some hotshot preacher who may not be the real deal.

Jesus declares to Nicodemus that if he has any chance of inheriting or entering the kingdom of God, he must be born again. Nicodemus ignorantly and innocently asks whether it's possible for a man of his age to reenter his mother's womb. I, too, was constantly stumped by the phrase *born again* until I began to focus on the details surrounding Nicodemus's initial birth. I couldn't crack the code concerning Jesus's mysterious words until I stumbled upon this Jewish prayer that would have been recited by religious Jewish males during the time of Jesus:

Blessed are you, Hashem, King of the Universe, for not having made me a Gentile.

Blessed are you, Hashem, King of the Universe, for not having made me a slave.

Blessed are you, Hashem, King of the Universe, for not having made me a woman.

Nicodemus was born a Jew, Nicodemus was born free, and Nicodemus was born male. Daily, he would have thanked God for his Jewishness, his freedom, and his gender, and he had built his life, reputation, and sense of self and identity on those three things. And that's why Jesus declares that Nicodemus must be *born again* in order to inherit the kingdom of God.

The kingdom identity isn't built on ethnicity. In God's kingdom, status isn't contingent on any social totem pole created by humans, and gender doesn't determine power or privilege. So Jesus is adamant that all the advantages and privileges Nicodemus was born with will not ultimately help him enter God's kingdom. In fact, because Nicodemus places so much value on his social status, it's become more of a barrier to true identity formation than a blessing. For his entire life, Nicodemus has been brain washed by a broken social system to regard his gender, freedom, and ethnicity as the foundation of his identity. If he chooses to be born again and enter into the kingdom of God, he must surrender all the broken pieces of identity he's built his life on thus far.

This doesn't apply only to Nicodemus. If we are going to enter the kingdom of God, we must stop placing our trust in and building our identity around elements of our first birth. Rather, we must trust and build around the elements of our *re*birth.

God loves the creativity and beauty expressed in our differences. Moreover, our differences are the artistic work of an imaginative God. He is pleased with the diversity and differences found within ethnicity, language, gender, and culture. Nothing we receive at birth, however, will be a sufficient substitute for building true identity. Only one identity marker matters for a born-again believer, and that's the illustrious and esteemed status as a child of God. To be God's son or daughter must hold so much value in our hearts and minds that our ethnicity, gender, social status, and any other idol takes a back seat to true identity as a child of God.

Once we're aware of the daily prayer offered by men like Nicodemus, Paul's words in Galatians 3:28 become painfully relevant: "There is neither Jew nor Gentile, neither slave nor free, nor is there male and female, for you are all one in Christ Jesus." Paul brings up ethnicity, social status, and gender because those three elements of identity are common pitfalls for every human walking this planet. They were common traps for Paul's original audience, they were a common trap for Nicodemus and his religious friends, and they're a common trap for you and me as we attempt to build our identity upon the solid rock of our adoption as sons and daughters of God.

As long as we hold on to the identity markers we received at birth, we'll only be full of ourselves. But the moment we're brain washed by the Mind of Christ, believing that adoption as sons and daughters is the foundation of identity, we become filled with the

Holy Spirit of God. This is why the conversation with Nicodemus quickly becomes centered around the person of the Holy Spirit. Jesus says to Nicodemus in John 3:6–8,

> Flesh gives birth to flesh, but the Spirit gives birth to spirit. You should not be surprised at my saying, "You must be born again." The wind blows wherever it pleases. You hear its sound, but you cannot tell where it comes from or where it is going. So it is with everyone born of the Spirit.

My first birth was physical. My rebirth is spiritual. With the Mind of Adam, we've been brain washed to believe in priority of our first birth when Jesus is clear that once we're born again, our spiritual identity takes center stage and our flesh-centered identity markers become background vocalists, completely subservient to the Spirit of God.

Ethnicity

Race

Height

Gender

Status

Accomplishments

Sexual orientation

Jesus sums all this up as flesh.

Does your confidence come from your first birth or your second birth?

Does your status come from where you stand socially or where you're seated spiritually?

Does your allegiance follow the temporary traits of your flesh or the eternal nature of your adoption?

In modern-day church culture, when we say *born again*, we typically direct those words toward non-Christian folks to inspire conversion. But these words were originally spoken to a very religious Jewish man who represented the upper echelon of morality and purity. This inconsistency has forced me to wonder about and question the motivation behind Jesus's precise language of being "born again." Nicodemus is clearly confused by the statement, and honestly, I've always been confused by it as well. I'm afraid that we've watered down a powerful and life-changing phrase into churchy lingo and holy-roller jargon.

The unfortunate reality is that since Jesus spoke these words to Nicodemus, millions of people have "converted" to Christianity but still center their identity around their flesh, not their spirit. We've made being "born again" about conversion when really to be born again is a radical declaration that our identities are no longer centered around characteristics of the flesh but around our spiritual identity as children of God. Like Nicodemus, we can find ourselves busy with religious behaviors but still needing to be born again as God's sons and daughters.

Does your confidence come from what you inherited at birth from your biological parents? Do your insecurities come from what you inherited at birth from your biological parents? If the answer to either of those questions is yes, then you must be born again.

Jesus emphatically declares that our identity should come only from the spiritual inheritance we received at our rebirth from our spiritual Father. Imagine what God's church and world would look like if we walked in the power of true spiritual identity. Imagine what this world would look like if ethnicity, social status, and gender did not divide us.

God's original design was for us to live in a world where ethnicity, gender, and social status weren't protected as holy or worshiped as idols but simply appreciated and celebrated as expressions of God's creativity. Jesus gave His life for a world where ethnicity, gender, and social status would be neither badges of pride nor sources of shame. The kingdom Jesus invites us into is where the power of our identity comes from our rebirth rather than our birth. Paul envisions a world where there is neither Jew nor Gentile, neither slave nor free, nor male and female but where we are all one in Christ Jesus.

The world I'm describing isn't a color-blind or whitewashed world but one where adoption as God's sons and daughters fills our minds so powerfully that our ethnicity, social status, and gender become peripheral instead of central.

The recreated cosmos described in Revelation is a world where women don't have to fight to be valued. What if we lived in a world where neither femininity nor masculinity had to be protected or asserted? As Christians, we must imagine and then create a world where minority groups don't have to protest for their rights. The kingdom of God is a place where everyone enjoys the beauty of human diversity and differences. The kingdom of God established on this colony of heaven is possible only when our identity is rooted in our rebirth, not our first birth, and that world is exactly how our Father describes heaven.

That world is what God intended when He placed Adam in the garden of Eden. But the Mind of Adam has created a world where identity is found in ethnicity, gender, and social status. Nicodemus was a son of Adam, not a son of God, and I'm afraid that on a daily basis we trade our spiritual inheritance for our biological inheritance. When God looks down at His creation, He sees the sons and daughters of Adam fighting over petty differences while neglecting their crowns as His sons and daughters. Like children who would rather play with the gift-wrapping paper than the actual gifts, we have idolized the outer wrappings of our flesh and neglected the spiritual status God has given us through Christ.

Why would we ever settle for being white or black or female or male or rich or anything else when we could be sons and daughters of God?

Nicodemus and the apostle Paul have a lot in common. In the book of Philippians, Paul gives us a little background concerning his past. At first, in chapter 3, verse 4, he sounds like he's bragging, because he says "I myself have reasons for such confidence. If someone else thinks they have reasons to put confidence in the flesh, I have more." Then in verses 5–6, he lists seven really impressive reasons why he could have such confidence:

1. "circumcised on the eighth day"
2. "of the people of Israel"
3. "of the tribe of Benjamin"
4. "a Hebrew of Hebrews"
5. "in regard to the law, a Pharisee"
6. "as for zeal, persecuting the church"
7. "as for righteousness based on the law, faultless"

But then Paul throws a curveball and says that all these impressive accomplishments and accolades are garbage. Trash. Worthless.

His ethnicity?
His religion?
His nationality?
His entire first birth?
Garbage.

Paul admits that, before Christ, he was full of himself but that it meant nothing because all the accomplishments in the universe could never compare to his being known as a son of God. Paul was full of himself and empty, and only in admitting our emptiness will we ever be filled.

Paul's exact words are:

But whatever were gains to me I now consider loss for the sake of Christ. What is more, I consider everything a loss because of the surpassing worth of knowing Christ Jesus my Lord, for whose sake I have lost all things. I consider them garbage, that I may gain Christ. (Philippians 3:7–8)

Paul was brain washed.

Brain washed with the Mind of Christ.

Brain washed with new identity.

Brain washed and born again.

Like Nicodemus, Paul was a free Jewish male, and before his conversion to the way of Jesus, he would have prayed the exact same Jewish prayer offered up by Nicodemus. Paul's identity and sense of self-worth were previously based on his socioeconomic privilege, along with his maleness, followed by his Jewish heritage.

Knowing that men like Paul and Nicodemus would have thanked God for not allowing them to be born into slavery or as a Gentile or as a woman helps place Paul's words from Galatians 3:28 in the appropriate context: "There is neither Jew nor Gentile, neither slave nor free, nor is there male and female, for you are all one in Christ Jesus." Paul references all three categories from the prayer that Nicodemus, he, and countless other free Jewish men would have been reciting. Paul is declaring that those identity markers do not suffice for followers of Jesus who have been brain washed into their true identity.

Nicodemus and Paul both had a lot of stock invested in their original definitions of identity, and I think we can all relate to that. The longer we contemplate what we're sacrificing, though, the longer it will take to make the switch. Humans, like the animals, were created from the dirt, and everything based on our original definition of identity correlates to the "dirt" of our humanity. Race, gender, ethnicity, socioeconomic status, political affiliations, and professional achievements are all just different combinations of the same dirt. When we define ourselves based on these visible characteristics, we shortchange ourselves. When we value only our dirt, we forfeit the glory of true humanity and settle for living like animals.

But fortunately, our Creator didn't just leave us as dirt pods but breathed life into our nostrils, thereby changing our design, which inevitably changed the definitions we use for our identity. When God breathed life into our souls, we became His children, made in His image, ready to rule and designed to reflect His glory and righteousness.

The second-century church father Irenaeus declared that "the glory of God is man fully alive." Humanity can be fully alive only when we live from the power of our true identity, when we're convinced of who we really are. When God's children live in confident humility, they have the boldness to bring healing to a broken world, and that glorifies God. When image-bearers reflect God's presence, wisdom, and beauty into every sphere of life, God is glorified. When Christians are convinced of the good news, the world is set ablaze with the veracity of the gospel, and God is glorified.

I don't know what thoughts of self you've entertained in the past, but this chapter has been a labor of love to convince you that your self-critical or self-debasing thoughts have no grounds in the truth. Your low self-esteem doesn't glorify God. Your false humility doesn't glorify God. Neither does your shame, guilt, or self-condemnation. None of those trains of thought are destined for the glory of God.

The Greek word for repentance is *metanoiein* or μετάνοια (phonetically pronounced met-an'-oy-ah), and it's become the English word *metanoia*. It's a powerful compound word. The first part of the word, *meta*, means change. The second half, *noia*, comes from the word *mind*. Translated literally, the word means "repentance," and *Merriam-Webster Dictionary* defines *metanoia* as "a transformative change of heart."[3] I've discovered that, so often in church, we're led to believe that we're repenting when in reality we're simply regretting our actions, vowing to change, and promising God behavior modification. But God isn't looking for behavior modification or regret. He's looking for repentance, which is a change of mind and a heart transformation in how we process our thoughts.

If you think you're ugly, repent.

If you think you're a sinner, repent.

If you think you need to earn God's approval, repent.

If you can't see how you're uniquely gifted, repent.

If you think you're just dirt, repent.

If your thoughts are prideful, repent.

Pride is the sin of thinking about yourself in terms that are higher or lower than the definition God has placed on humanity. Pride is the sin of overvaluing or undervaluing yourself. Pride is ultimately a focus on self that manifests either in arrogance or low self-esteem. When we adopt God's identity for ourselves, we avoid both arrogance and low self-esteem, and we begin to walk in the power of confidence and humility. Confident, humble people secure in their identity are fully alive, bring glory to God, and are healthy and ready for rich interpersonal relationships—our last stop on the journey to adopting the Mind of Christ.

6

Designed for Connection

The LORD God said, "It is not good for the man to be alone."

Genesis 2:18

I USED TO GET ANNOYED at the very sight of Brian Bullock—that is, until we became best friends. All my other friends were shocked and nervous when I told them Brian and I had been hanging out and truly getting to know each other. They weren't prepared for me to abruptly end my constant and oftentimes verbal disapproval of him, and their emotional whiplash was visible by the confusion and concern written across their faces.

For years, I had perceived Brian as a gossiping, two-faced, disloyal, unfashionable opportunist, and I had a mountain of evidence in support of my opinion. But then I learned Brian had his own mountain of evidence in support of his negative opinion of *me*.

Things about Brian's personality definitely clashed with mine, but our insecurities clashed far more violently and way more frequently than our personalities. My thoughts about Brian were actually a reflection of how I thought about myself. Jealousy, comparison, and distrust are the natural by-products of an insecure mindset. The Mind of Christ is rooted in intimacy with the Father. The Mind of Christ is clear concerning identity. And finally, the Mind of Christ walks interdependently with others.

I felt like I was a child on a playdate planned by my parents when Brian and I stood in Pastor Andy's kitchen and got told to drop our petty grievances and disagreements and intentionally choose friendship. Clearly, our pastor could see what we couldn't. He explained that we had a unique opportunity to choose friendship, and that comparison and defensiveness could rob us of that opportunity.

I had responded to Brian's arrival on the scene like an only child who's just found out his parents are pregnant. It marked the end of my monopoly on attention and resources. I grew up in Boston, and I remember the feeling of anticipation in the air when ballplayer David Ortiz would step up to the plate, especially in the post season. Everyone knew what was about to happen. Red Sox fans knew. Ortiz's teammates knew. The opposing team knew. We had all seen him hit homers, and we knew this time would be no different. When Brian stepped on stage to preach or sing, it was like that. (It's still like that. The only difference is that now I'm a supporter and a fan, not an insecure critic.)

Not until years later did Brian and I realize that we had admired each other more than we'd disliked each other. My journey of friendship with him has taught me that jealousy and comparison will cause you to compete and gossip when you should be learning and befriending.

Pastor Andy perceived that we had the opportunity to relate to each other based on our commonalities but could also challenge each other to grow. He perceived that a friendship, like braces on teeth, would bring correction to our souls despite initial pain and discomfort. He perceived that many shepherds choose the safety of solely relating to sheep and avoid other shepherds. And he perceived that leaders can quite naturally be loners, but that by doing so, we deny our nature and defy our original design as humans.

My friendship with Brian taught me that we often confuse that which is foreign for that which is flawed.

I'll never forget our first moment of raw honesty. Brian admitted that he found me to be arrogant and self-absorbed. This was the first honest thing I had heard him say, and his critique of my behavior and character was the beginning of our friendship.

The first time Brian made me log into my online banking and show him my transaction history was uncomfortable. He added up how much I'd spent on fast food. The discomfort wasn't a sign of dysfunction but rather growing pains. When he called me for the first time to tell me that he'd livestreamed a Sunday service and found my sermon to be subpar, I was also uncomfortable. But I learned that when iron starts to sharpen iron, sparks fly. My friendship with Brian forced me to confront my own insecurities and caused me to begin building and fortifying my true identity. And the only way to form my true identity was to become intimate with God, which exposed my ideas concerning Him.

This means the journey you and I have been on for chapters now is actually a loop. The journey from independence to intimacy, from insecurity to identity, and from isolation to interdependence can be entered at any of the three stages. Ideas about God will inevitably inform our ideas about self and others, yet it's also true that ideas about others inevitably expose our ideas concerning self and ultimately God. This three-way, looped relationship is deeply interconnected.

The human ego is great at protecting us from the kind of emotional nudity I felt as Brian and I became friends. God originally created Adam as a lone wolf. He was made in the image of God as the pinnacle of creation, but he had nobody to relate to, only creatures to lead. (A short note to leaders: Notice that Adam was placed in positional leadership over creation, but God observed that he had relationships only with beings who could not challenge him. So He declared this state of affairs to be detrimental. As long as you relate only to those whom you lead, you are effectively alone. Loneliness and isolation are both riskier than the challenge of friendship.)

There's no stronger or more accurate litmus test for insecurity than the quality and nature of our interpersonal relationships. Our ideas of others are truly a reflection of our thoughts concerning ourselves. Conversely, there's no faster vehicle for correcting an insecure soul than healthy interdependent relationships.

Relationships reveal whether comparison, distrust, jealousy, defensiveness, passive-aggressive patterns, emotional neediness, and a proclivity toward being easily offended exist in our soul. Those are all symptoms that point to inner sickness, and they can be ignored, masked, or addressed. My prayer is that this chapter will cause you to stop and think about your relationships and then address the underlying causes of any sickness with the appropriate method of healing.

Brian Bullock and I pushed through the discomfort and vulnerability of our newly mandated friendship, and I'm glad we did. The result has been a life-giving oasis of truth, forgiveness, wisdom, and hope, and the journey left me with indispensable lessons on the brokenness of human relationship and the wholeness Jesus offers as we choose to let Him brain wash us and rewire our minds.

I'm convinced that the Serpent had always been scared that one day Brian and I would begin to trust each other and become brothers. He knows humans were designed for intimacy, relationship, and community. Therefore, his technique for destroying humanity is to divide and conquer. Isolation and loneliness are kryptonite to the human soul, and nothing leads to isolation more quickly than an insecure thought process. Toxic thought patterns concerning others puts a strain on human relationships that leave us isolated and easy prey for the Serpent.

Giants and Grasshoppers

My friendship with Brian reminds me of something the children of Israel said at the conclusion of their forty-day exploration of Canaan. Numbers 13:27 records that the land God had promised to give them was indeed fruitful and desirable. But their own insecurities colored and tainted the way they saw God's blessing. Joshua and Caleb returned from Canaan with a positive report, believing God that He would work through them to bring about their victory. But the other ten spies spread fear among the people, saying, "We seemed like grasshoppers in our own eyes, and we looked the same to them" (Numbers 13:33).

I cringe while reading their words because the statement is fully infected with insecure thinking. For starters, they seemed like grasshoppers in their own eyes. They didn't see the identity God had declared over them but rather relied on how they felt about themselves. More importantly for the focus of this chapter, though, how they saw themselves had a major impact on how they thought about others. They close their sentence by saying "and we looked the same to them."

Here are two practical steps we can take.

Don't make assumptions.

The Israelites made an assumption regarding how other people viewed them. Insecurities don't just stop once they've achieved the goal of getting us to think negatively about ourselves. They seek to isolate us. They cause us to make assumptions about how others perceive us—and in my experience, the assumptions are rarely accurate. Did these spies perform interviews with the giants in question? Certainly not. They viewed themselves as grasshoppers and assumed everyone else saw them according to the same pattern. Insecurities always lead to assumptions and false conclusions.

I love that the Bible eventually solves this mystery, telling us exactly how the inhabitants of Canaan really saw the Israelites. In the second chapter of Joshua, Rahab tells the spies they were never seen as grasshoppers. On the contrary, she says,

> "I know that the LORD has given you this land and that a great fear of you has fallen on us, so that all who live in this country are melting in fear because of you. We have heard how the LORD dried up the water of the Red Sea for you when you came out of Egypt, and what you did to Sihon and Og, the two kings of the Amorites east of the Jordan, whom you completely destroyed. When we heard of it, our hearts melted in fear and everyone's courage failed because of you, for the LORD your God is God in heaven above and on the earth below." (Joshua 2:9–11)

The giants the Israelites were afraid of were themselves afraid. The giants didn't see the Israelites as grasshoppers at all. The Israelites were completely wrong, and I have personally stopped drawing thought bubbles above everyone's head and assuming what they think. I've been wrong too many times. And so have you.

Somehow, our insecurities convince us that we have psychic power, but we don't. Thankfully, we don't know what's happening in the minds of other people. Neither do we know their motives. If we're going to move from isolation to interdependence, we must stop assuming we know the minds and motives of others. The Mind of Adam makes assumptions. It's marked by the questions found in Matthew 16, where Jesus asks, "Who do people say the Son of Man is?" (verse 13) and "Who do you say I am?" (verse 15).

If you really want to know what people think of you, don't assume. Simply ask. Insecure people make assumptions. People who are brain washed to be secure in their identity are constantly seeking counsel and critique so they can improve and become more self-aware. Insecure people tend not to ask others difficult questions because they're scared of the answers and are prone to being easily offended.

If you want to take practical steps toward becoming more confident, then you must stop making assumptions concerning the minds and motives of others. When we make assumptions about how others perceive us or about their motives concerning us, we become paranoid. And paranoia is emotionally expensive.

Seek input.

A second practical step is to then seek out some critique from a handful of people you trust. Assure them that you will not be offended by what they say, nor will you allow their compliments to make you proud. This kind of honesty and safety has been the greatest gift of my friendship with Brian. Proverbs 27:6 teaches us that "wounds from a friend can be trusted, but an enemy multiplies kisses." We would be wise to accept this counterintuitive wisdom from Solomon. When we seek out critique, and someone we trust tells us about an area that can use improvement, it wounds our ego, and compliments and flattery are like kisses. Solomon makes it clear that a good friend won't hold back the blade of truth, and that a secure person won't cut off relationship when the blade gets pulled out.

As noted earlier, in John 15 Jesus describes Himself as the true vine that gives life to everything connected to Him. The Father is described as a meticulous gardener who carefully tends to humanity and the individual soul. The passage is beautiful and encouraging as Jesus promises us, "If you remain in me and I in you, you will bear much fruit" (verse 5). This passage is full of intimate language and the promise of fruitfulness. But it's also dark and gloomy, because in verse 2 Jesus says, "[The Father] cuts off every branch in me that bears no fruit, while every branch that does bear fruit he prunes so that it will be even more fruitful."

This is a double dose of bad news. A lack of fruitfulness leads to being cut. Fruitfulness also leads to being cut. There's no way to avoid the blades of God's pruning shears, and I have learned that oftentimes my friend Brian was being held in the hands of God like a blade to cut and prune my pride so I could bear even more fruit.

Insecure thinking not only kept me from befriending Brian for several years but nearly robbed me of marrying the wife of my dreams. And again, Pastor Andy was the fateful bearer of uncomfortable truth.

He had met Tia and come to the conclusion everyone else who met her had come to as well. She was beautiful, smart, witty, and gifted, and she loved Jesus and had a clear call to ministry. We got along great, rarely argued, and had an incredible friendship. So Pastor Andy asked me, "Manny, why haven't you married Tia? Why do you seem so *on the fence* about her? What's wrong with the girl?"

I'd known Pastor Andy since the age of eleven, so I felt comfortable being honest. "I don't like that she's taller than me."

As if he didn't even need time to process my response, he immediately said, "I asked you what was wrong with her, not what was wrong with you. Her height isn't the problem. *Your* height is the problem. And your height is only a problem to you. That's an insecurity."

I had no words.

I barely had breath.

I sank into the back seat of the rental car we were in, and "I never thought about it that way" was the most sophisticated response I could muster.

His next comment cut even deeper. "Manny, you're five foot five, right? Here's the deal. If you marry someone who's five foot two, you'll still be five foot five. If you marry someone who's five foot nine, you'll still be five foot five, and nothing will ever change that. Moreover, your height doesn't matter. You're gifted, and you're anointed. When you preach, people's lives are changed. When you're on stage preaching and people are getting set free, they aren't secretly wishing you were taller. Nobody cares about your height but you. Nobody thinks about your height but you. Just focus on your strengths and forget about your height."

I was engaged to Tia two months later.

I had been making a toxic assumption. I assumed that people saw me the same way I saw myself. I assumed that being short affected how people respected, esteemed, or treated me. The reality is that I was the only person who cared, but like the children of Israel declared in Numbers 13:33, I seemed like a grasshopper in my own eyes, and I thought I looked the same to everyone else.

The best gift you could give yourself is the gift of relationship with an emotionally inexpensive person. Becoming emotionally inexpensive means you can give others the gift of relationship as well, which results in healthy interdependence.

Insecure thinking makes us emotionally expensive and exhausting, but when we walk in the power of our identity as a child of God, we begin to flourish and grow the fruit of confidence and humility. True confidence and humility are the marks of emotionally healthy people. They become the jet fuel that empowers us to escape the gravitational pull of both independence and codependence. Only then do we have the freedom to choose interdependent relationships, which is God's design for humans.

Paralysis, Pools, and Peers

Two particular paralyzed men stand out to me when I read the account of Jesus's life in the Gospels. The first man isn't a stranger on our journey because we talked about him at length back in chapter 3. He was the man who sat beside the pool at Bethesda all day. But the second paralyzed man makes his debut in this chapter, and he has a valuable lesson to teach us as we pilgrimage from the Mind of Adam to the Mind of Christ.

Mark 2:3 says, "Some men came, bringing to [Jesus] a paralyzed man, carried by four of them." The first striking thing about this story is that this paralyzed man wasn't at the pool of Bethesda, where paralyzed persons had their own section and Jesus found our other paralyzed pilgrim. Instead of hanging out at the famous pool with other paralyzed people, this man in Mark 2 had made friends with people who could walk.

The second detail I find striking is that more than four friends brought him to Jesus. Mark says, "some men came," and that he was carried by "four" of them. Maybe six or seven men brought this paralytic to Jesus. Perhaps it was twelve or fifteen. We don't know the exact number, but we do know the man had enough relational equity that a group of his friends didn't mind carrying him to the house where Jesus was, ripping up a roof, and then lowering him inside. That's impressive, because most paralyzed people would not have had that same relational equity.

Most paralyzed people hung out with other paralyzed people.

Most paralyzed people felt the most comfortable at the pool of Bethesda.

But here we find a paralyzed man with a large group of non-paralyzed friends who care about him, and that's peculiar because I can only imagine how emotionally challenging it would be to watch your friends walk around all day knowing that you can't. There's a reason all the paralyzed people formed a congregation at the pool; it was their comfort zone, there was relatability, and there was comfort. I applaud this man for the courage it took to choose to be around people who could walk instead. Already I can tell he's not insecure, because the sight of walking would make an insecure person wallow in self-pity and feel self-conscious.

When I was younger, I desperately wished my dad was more normal or traditional. Because of his addiction, he was always in and out of our home, and he didn't teach me how to change a tire or pick out a suit. So whenever I was around my friends who had amazing fathers, jealousy, resentment, and comparison rose up within my heart and mind. Being around the very thing I longed for was a trigger for my insecurities. That's why I'm shocked that this paralyzed man deliberately surrounded himself with people who could walk around freely. And this single decision pays off when these friends use their ability and collective compassion to take the man to Jesus.

Do you remember what the man from the pool of Bethesda said? When Jesus asked him if he wanted to be healed, his knee-jerk response was, "I have no one to help me" (John 5:7). Well, go figure. How could anyone help you when everyone at the pool is in the same condition you are? How could anyone help you when you've chosen to surround yourself with people who make you feel comfortable? There's no growth in our comfort zones, and for most people their comfort zone represents their circle of closest friendships.

Here are two approaches you can take toward confidence and interdependence when you're paralyzed.

Surround yourself with those who are strong where you are weak.

Help is readily available when you surround yourself with people who are strong where you are weak. I finally stopped allowing healthy paternal relationship to be a trigger for me and started learning from surrogate and spiritual fathers. I've learned about fatherhood from placing myself around great fathers and watching them in action. Whereas before my insecurities isolated me and relegated me to my own proverbial Pool of Wounded and Neglected Sons—where I, too, had "no one to help me"—now I count my friends with great fathers as a blessing.

The irony of the man at the pool of Bethesda is that Jesus is standing right there with the power to help and heal. But when we choose isolation, we're trained to make assumptions about the minds and motives of others, which is a waste of emotional energy. The man at the pool clearly didn't assume that Jesus was there to help; oftentimes people with issues assume they're a burden. But not our friend being carried by his friends. He has none of the mental hang-ups evident in our other paralyzed friend.

Both men were paralyzed, and they both ended up healed. But they made radically different decisions about who to surround themselves with, what assumptions would guide their thinking, and how they felt about themselves.

Be around people who can do what you can't do.

Another practical step toward confidence and interdependence is to surround yourself with people who trigger your insecurities and then overcome those insecurities. Get around people who can do what you can't do. Most likely God is trying to bless you with a friendship that will elevate your thinking, but your insecurities are keeping you jealous, resentful, and bitter.

If you want to earn a million dollars, surround yourself with millionaires. Yes, drive your Honda Civic and park it right next to a millionaire's Maserati, swallow your pride, and choose your relationship with wisdom, not your feelings. If you want to be married, hang out with married people. Yes, you may be the awkward third wheel, or fifth wheel, or twenty-seventh wheel, but eventually someone will bring their single cousin around, and you may end up liking them.

My wife and I welcomed a son in 2021, but we struggled with infertility for years. During that time, we desperately wanted to be parents, so we babysat for our friends who had kids. We helped plan baby showers, and we also waited with anticipation at multiple gender reveal parties. We could have easily become bitter, but instead we allowed our "non-paralyzed" friends to build our faith.

I was a pretty amazing kid . . . so I'm told. I started talking early, and my parents can attest that once they bought me big-boy underwear with my beloved Teenage Mutant Ninja Turtles screenprinted on the back, I was immediately potty-trained. I wouldn't dare disrespect Donatello, Michelangelo, Raphael, or Leonardo like that.

Most importantly, especially for my street cred, I started walking very young. My cousin, however, was not so eager to get off his belly and put an end to the crawling. He was well past his first birthday and still wasn't walking, and although I was the oldest, we were only weeks apart in age. Then my parents had a genius idea. They told my aunt to bring him to our house so he could be around someone his age who was mobile and killing the game. My parents claimed that adults aren't good at motivating kids to walk, but being in the presence of other little people could be just the trick.

So my aunt dropped off my cousin to spend a week with us. Soon he and I were running around our cramped inner-city apartment, and he had ditched crawling altogether.

I've learned that sometimes God places an "older cousin" in your life who can easily perform the task you long to accomplish, and your insecurities will determine whether you choose isolation or interdependence. My prayer is that you won't let your insecurities keep you paralyzed.

Why did this group of guys care so much about their paralyzed friend receiving supernatural healing? And why didn't this man see himself as a burden? I'm going to make an assumption: I think it was because he was an incredible friend.

What if your paralyzed friend gave such good advice that you felt indebted to him? What if your paralyzed friend was a constant source of encouragement? What if your paralyzed friend covered you and your family in prayer every single day? What if your paralyzed friend knew his worth and value and didn't see himself as a burden but a blessing?

Then you would gladly want to repay your friend for everything he's done for you. Maybe the paralyzed guy knew he could help his town more than he could help other paralyzed people at a pool. Maybe the paralyzed guy was secure, full of identity, and enjoyed intimacy with the Father. Maybe the paralyzed guy was brain washed.

Just because you're paralyzed doesn't mean you have nothing to offer. The only thing that will keep you from offering what God has placed within you is seeing yourself as a grasshopper instead of the giant you really are.

I believe these guys brought their friend to Jesus because they were in a healthy, reciprocal, interdependent relationship with him. My prayer is that you will choose that kind of relationship for yourself as well.

Now let's explore the beauty of true interdependence.

What Is Interdependence?

Interdependence was God's original design for human relationship, but unfortunately the Serpent drives us toward isolation using two vehicles of choice: codependence and independence. Let's unpack both.

My parents spent thirty years of life in a codependent relationship, so I know firsthand how toxic they can be. When they met, my mother was trapped in a dysfunctional relationship with a physically abusive husband who had raped and consistently beat her. My dad had a need to be needed, so one day he attacked her abusive husband, beat him up pretty bad, and proceeded to move my mother into his home.

My father abused drugs but was the breadwinner for the family and used his ability to provide financially as relational leverage. My mother was physically disabled and was able to qualify for government-assisted housing. After one of his drug binges, my mother would nurse my dad back to strength, and he would continue to bring home the bacon.

They each provided something the other couldn't provide for themselves. They took turns being codependent, and that cycle was toxic for our family.

My dad wasn't happy but didn't want to be homeless.

My mom wasn't happy but didn't want to be poor.

My dad was indispensable because of his income.

My mom was indispensable because of her apartment.

They both took advantage of the situation. My dad got to live in a nice warm home with a wife who cared enough to cook, clean, and help him appear respectable. My dad needed my mom, and my mom needed to be needed. My father was dependent on my mom, and my mother was codependent on him. Codependency is a vicious cycle.

Codependence is fueled by the fear of being alone, without love and practical resources. The sad reality is that codependent relationships can't produce true intimacy because they lack honesty, transparency, and unconditional acceptance.

My parents lived in the same home, but they were both lonely and isolated. My dad kept secrets and was in constant hiding. My mom found value only in what she could do, never in who she was, but performing for love is not intimacy. Codependency creates arrangements between people, not intimate relationship.

Those who are repulsed by toxic codependent cycles typically opt for the extreme opposite relational dysfunction. Yet that pattern still ends at the same destination, which is isolation. Same destination, different vehicle.

The opposite of codependency is total independence, which is also rooted in fear. People attempt to walk through life without meeting or admitting their natural human need for love, intimacy, and connection. Independence is a toxic lie, because humans are relational beings God designed for connection and intimacy. People who opt for independence are operating under the deception that it's possible to tackle life alone. That's understandable if you're paranoid about falling into the ditch of codependent relational dysfunction. We must realize, though, that there's a ditch on both sides of this narrow road toward the Mind of Christ, and His model for human relationship isn't codependence or independence but rather interdependence.

Let's talk more about being emotionally inexpensive and how being emotionally *expensive* leads to isolation. Intimacy with God and a healthy understanding of self makes us emotionally inexpensive, and people will love being around us. Insecure thoughts drive us toward comparison and jealousy, which are toxic relational structures that end in isolation. Thoughts of low self-esteem drive us to demand validation from others, which makes us emotionally expensive and drives us toward isolation. A constant need for affirmation will make us toxic and manipulative in an effort to control those around us, which, again, will inevitably end in isolation.

People secure in their identity aren't needy. People full of God's brain washed identity don't require human applause because they've received heaven's approval. When people walk with God intimately and receive identity from Him and truly love and accept themselves, they're emotionally inexpensive for the people surrounding them, and they become easy to love.

The greatest gift you could possibly give your closest friends and family is the gift of a low-maintenance relationship. This is the gift Jesus gave to all those whom He called His closest friends. The Serpent robbed Adam and Eve of their God-given design for interdependence, but Jesus modeled humanity for us so that we no longer must walk in the fallen footsteps of Adam and Eve.

Interdependence is the understanding that although humans need connection and intimacy, that need is never to be exploited or taken advantage of. Interdependence can exist only between two healthy individuals who are walking in intimacy with God and receiving their identity from Him. Interdependence requires mental health and wholeness, and in turn it produces mental health and wholeness. Isolation is prompted by toxic mindsets and perpetuates those same toxic mindsets.

Jesus was a model for interdependence, and the Mind of Christ is marked by a refusal to settle for the extremes of independence and isolation. This may seem simple, but I really enjoy the fact that Jesus had friends. The Bible records that He went to Bethany often because His friends lived there and their house was His favorite place to laugh, relax, and eat good food. Yes, even Jesus had relational needs, which means none of us are getting accolades from Him by denying *our* relational needs. Jesus is the model and blueprint for how to be truly human, and He thoroughly enjoyed hanging out with Mary, Martha, and Lazarus.

Denying their relational needs doesn't make anyone more spiritual. So often in church I hear people say things like, "I just need to focus on my relationship with God." Or even worse, "All I need is Jesus." Nothing could be further from the truth. Remember when God created Adam and they had infinite amounts of one-on-one time with no distractions? That wasn't an ideal humans fell from. God declared that this wasn't enough, so He rebooted the creation machine and gave Adam the gift of *human* relationship. Therefore, God isn't "enough" or "the only thing we need," and that's amazing. Our infinitely wise Creator made us with an indispensable need for intimate relationship with Him *and* others.

Jesus models this beautifully. In Luke 10, He's at His favorite house with His favorite people, and like always, Martha is cooking. I can completely relate to Jesus's love of food. He's made really good wine and even miraculously multiplied fish sandwiches. He's miraculously made fish appear so that Peter could catch them. Even death couldn't stop Jesus from eating. After His resurrection, He appears to His crew of frightened disciples, shows them His crucifixion scars, and then immediately lightens the mood by asking them for some food.

If you don't find that story of Jesus downright hilarious, then you may be reading the Bible wrong. Jesus also invites Himself to eat the wealthy cuisine at Zacchaeus's house, and to be honest, we find Jesus at dinner tables often. Jesus was a foodie, and that made Martha's place perfect. He could tell Lazarus and Mary the latest outrageous remark Peter made and grab some of Martha's incredible cooking at the same time.

But Jesus wasn't interested in relational dysfunction.

> *If you're doing this because you need to be needed, Martha, then stop.*
>
> *If you think your cooking makes you important to Me, then stop.*
>
> *If you said yes verbally but your heart says no, then stop.*
>
> *If you think I just see you as a cook, then stop.*
>
> *Martha, I care more about you than your food, so stop.*

Jesus wanted no part of any codependent cycle. He would rather hear a true and honest no than a false or disingenuous yes. Some of us have toxic relationships because we take advantage of other people's verbal yes even when we know they mean no in their heart. Some of us have toxic relationships because we don't know how to say no, and the Mind of Christ can't be formed within us until we reject relational dysfunction. Jesus doesn't take advantage of anyone, and neither should we. Jesus had real needs, but only willing hearts were allowed to meet those needs.

Jesus's commitment to healthy interpersonal dynamics can be clearly seen in another story with the same cast of characters: Lazarus, Mary, and Martha. John 11:3 records that "the sisters sent word to Jesus, 'Lord, the one you love is sick.'"

I love the subtle reminder these women give Jesus. They don't just say, "Lazarus is sick, and we need You to heal him." Instead, they remind Jesus that He loves Lazarus. We must read between the lines here. The sisters are essentially saying, "Since You've said You love our brother, Lazarus, it would be nice for You to put that love in action and heal him. Please and thank You, Jesus."

That reading isn't simple literary license but consistent with what we know about Martha's personality. In Luke 10, Martha has shown us that she tends to be the kind of person who will do what you ask even if she doesn't necessarily want to. To be honest, Martha sounds like a classic 2 on the Enneagram. People who battle with saying no also use favors as leverage for what they may need in the future.

Someone like Martha could be thinking to herself, *OK, Lazarus is sick. I'm so glad I cooked all those meals for Jesus. Now I can cash in a favor, and Jesus can heal Lazarus. Jesus kind of owes us one anyway. He's always here, and I always cook and never ask for anything in return. Plus, He said He really loves Lazarus.*

Now, I don't know Martha, but I know my own heart, and I know these thoughts would have floated through my mind. If you're honest, you'll admit they may have floated through your mind as well.

Jesus didn't take advantage of people, and in this story we'll soon learn He didn't allow anyone to emotionally manipulate Him either. Thousands of sermons and books have been preached and written on the raising of Lazarus from the dead, but my goal isn't to add to any of them. This isn't about the resurrection; it's about the relationship Jesus had with this family. And moreover, it's about the relationships we have.

Jesus doesn't respond to Mary and Martha the way anyone would have expected. He does love them, and He specifically loves Lazarus, but He doesn't allow anyone to cash in favors with Him. John 11:5–6 records that "Jesus loved Martha and her sister and Lazarus. So when he heard that Lazarus was sick, he stayed where he was two more days." Jesus loves Lazarus, and He could leave right away to save him, but He doesn't because He isn't under any compulsion to prove His love.

Jesus certainly demonstrates love freely, but He doesn't respond to any perceived obligation to prove His love for us. John the Baptist tried to pull the Get-Your-Cousin-Out-of-Jail Card, and that didn't go over so well (Luke 7:18–22). And Jesus felt no pressure to prove to Satan that He was truly the Son of God (Luke 4:1–13). But He did demonstrate and communicate His identity to those who believed.

Whenever we find ourselves having to prove our love, we could be stuck in an unhealthy or emotionally exhaustive or codependent relationship cycle.

Jesus finally decides to go to Bethany, but by the time He arrives, Lazarus is already dead, and both sisters send Jesus on a pretty scenic guilt trip. John 11:21 records, "'Lord,' Martha said to Jesus, 'if you had been here, my brother would not have died.'"

Ouch.

Next, here comes Mary. John 11:32 says, "When Mary reached the place where Jesus was and saw him, she fell at his feet and said, 'Lord, if you had been here, my brother would not have died.'"

That sounds familiar.

I find it striking that Jesus doesn't respond to either sister. Nor does He entertain comments about His love for Lazarus, His timing, His motives, or what "coulda woulda shoulda" happened had He shown up as soon as they'd requested He come. It's as if Jesus doesn't even hear their emotionally manipulative statements. I've learned from Dr. Henry Cloud that no attention can be given to people who are emotionally manipulative. Reading his classic book *Boundaries*, coauthored with Dr. John Townsend, was a huge game changer for me.

Jesus avoided the toxic pitfall of codependence, but He also refused to live in the vacuum of isolation in the form of independence. The Trinity exists within the beauty of interdependence, and Jesus settled for nothing less while on Earth. He exhibited vulnerability, honesty, and relational courage. If anyone could have managed being a lone ranger, it would have certainly been Jesus. But even the most powerful human to ever live admitted a need for friendship, family, and intimacy.

Jesus's need for others can be observed clearly in the garden of Gethsemane. Matthew 26:38–40 describes the scene:

> [Jesus] said to them, "My soul is overwhelmed with sorrow to the point of death. Stay here and keep watch with me." Going a little farther, he fell with his face to the ground and prayed, "My Father, if it is possible, may this cup be taken from me. Yet not as I will, but as you will." Then he returned to his disciples and found them sleeping. "Couldn't you men keep watch with me for one hour?" he asked Peter.

Jesus asked for His disciples' presence, and He communicated this beautifully simple request by saying, "Stay here and keep watch with Me." Jesus is at the most stressful and overwhelming point of His life and makes a request that should help us redefine what we think we need from others.

Unfortunately, Peter and the crew fail to meet this basic need of presence. They simply can't stay awake, and the disappointment in Jesus's voice leaps off the page and pierces your soul when you read, "Couldn't you men keep watch with me for one hour?" (Matthew 26:40). The disciples fell short by failing to do more.

It's equally unfortunate that Job's friends fail to give him the same precious gift: their presence. Instead, they give him advice, theological arguments, explanations, and condemnation. His friends fall short by doing too much.

You may fall into any of the following four categories. If you do, the goal is to let the Mind of Christ brain wash you into being emotionally inexpensive for others.

1. Do you require too much from people? (Martha)
2. Do you give too much to people? (Martha and Job's friends)
3. Do you require too little from people? (Paralyzed man at the pool)
4. Do you give too little to people? (Peter and other disciples)

Not only does Jesus request the presence of His disciples and friends, but He promises and commits to giving them the same in return. He promises His presence when He declares, "Surely I am with you always, to the very end of the age" (Matthew 28:20).

Jesus also requests prayers, which He hoped for in Gethsemane.

In the garden, Jesus prays for His disciples and intercedes on our behalf to God the Father. Paul declares in Romans 8:34, "Who then is the one who condemns? No one. Christ Jesus who died—more than that, who was raised to life—is at the right hand of God and is also interceding for us."

We currently have the presence of Jesus and the prayers of Jesus, and although He isn't currently in emotional agony, He still needs the same two things from us that He requested of His disciples. Jesus's gift of His presence means nothing if we don't reciprocate, and an intercessor can only intercede based on the requests sent.

Interdependence demands that we give our presence and prayers to Jesus and to others. All the fruit of relational intimacy flows from those two basic needs. Jesus healed people because they were in His presence, and He prayed. He preached the truth in love and with authority because they were in His presence, and He prayed for the crowds. Like Martha, you may think you need many things, but when we first meet the sisters in Luke 10, Mary proves that only her presence is necessary. This is what Jesus asked for when He told Martha, "Mary has chosen what is better," and we would be wise to follow His lead.

Jesus didn't have hang-ups about asking the disciples to meet His needs. He wasn't too insecure, full of Himself, or too proud to make His needs known to His closest followers, whom He referred to as friends. He also didn't manipulate them or hit them with a guilt trip once they failed. The relational patterns of our Messiah must be modeled so that our relationships are life-giving and not draining. That starts with repenting of how we've thought about relationships.

Rat Park

My father has been a drug addict ever since I can remember, so I wish I had known about Rat Park sooner. Maybe as a family we could have supported him better. We all have assumptions and pre-determined opinions about drug addicts, especially those of us who grow up with one. But recently I've reshaped my opinions regarding addiction based on some eye-opening research and a fascinating TED Talk by Johann Hari titled "Everything You Think You Know About Addiction Is Wrong."[1]

The popular opinion is that those who are addicted have developed a physical dependency on the chemicals associated with their drug of choice. But in his 2015 TED Talk, Hari pointed out that if addiction is the result of exposure and chemical dependency, we'd have countless more addicts in the world. Why? Because many of us have been exposed to drugs, such as for pain after surgery, and never become addicts.

That means addiction is more complex than we may think, and unlocking the mystery could help us in our journey toward adopting the Mind of Christ.

This idea about drug addiction is more complex than I explain it here, so I invite you to listen to Hari's TED Talk for yourself. But here's what I learned through his talk and other sources. The conventional approach to viewing drug addiction is based on a set of experiments in the early twentieth century where both normal water and water with drugs in it were placed in the cages of individual lab rats who had nothing to do and no other being to relate to except the researchers who tended them. Those isolated rats came to prefer the drugged water, eventually killing themselves, thus the belief that drug dependency comes from the drug itself. But then Dr. Bruce Alexander and his colleagues conducted a series of experiments, and something mind-boggling took place.[2]

They created a cage they called a Rat Park, and inside, rather than isolating rats, they placed them with other rats of both sexes, gave them food as well as both plain and drugged water, and even gave them balls and wheels to play with. The result was that the rats did not prefer the drugged water, and they thrived. The researchers concluded that isolation versus community seemed to have made the difference, and observations made on humans exposed to drugs without becoming addicts have sparked the same idea that human drug addiction could be more about isolation than about drugs.

Rat Park isn't the most revolutionary part of this new perspective on addiction. In 2001, Portugal decided to decriminalize drug use and use the money they'd spent on cutting off addicts with isolation punishment to instead reconnect them with society. For instance, they established programs for job creation and business microloans for addicts who need them.

Whatever your opinion about decriminalizing drugs, my point is to take note of the effect this new policy seems to have had on Portugal's drug problem. So many people believe they need a miracle from God, but what if He intends for us to be one another's miracle?

A 2015 study found that since the Portugal Drug Policy was introduced, drug misuse decreased by 18%.

The percentage of people in prison in Portugal for drug law violations decreased dramatically from 44% in 1999 to 24% in 2013.

Between 1998 and 2011, the number of people in drug treatment programmes had increased by over 60%.[3]

I believe the Serpent was aware of how desperately humans need connection, intimacy, and community. If our theology only connects us back to God, it's incomplete. The Serpent severed Adam and

Eve from a life-giving relationship with God, but he also separated them from each other. They put fig leaves on to hide from God and each other, and relational strife exponentially increased. Within one generation, we had the first murder. The goal of the second Adam—Christ—is to reconnect humanity to God as well as one another, which is why God reverses the division of Babel at Pentecost. The Serpent's goal was to force Adam and Eve into isolation from each other, but Jesus lived so we could all reconnect.

Toward the beginning of this book, I mapped out three categories of thoughts over which we can and should have authority. All toxic thoughts can be organized into these three categories:

1. Thoughts about God
2. Thoughts about self
3. Thoughts about others

The Serpent attacks us with negative thoughts about God to separate us from our loving Father. He attacks us with negative thoughts about ourselves to keep us insecure and at odds with our own self. And he attacks us with negative thoughts about others to keep us isolated, alone, and disconnected. But we can overcome our negative thoughts so we can form lasting bonds that will produce peace, joy, and human flourishing.

If connection is a potential cure for addiction, then I have a sneaking suspicion that human connection has the power to cure the mindsets that sabotage our futures. Connection has the potential to lift loved ones out of a depressive mindset. Intimacy with others can break the mental strongholds of pessimism, negativity, and defeat.

The Mind of Christ propels us toward establishing strong relational bonds with others, and the bonds we form with others drive us deeper into the Mind of Christ.

Scrolling Is Emotionally and Spiritually Carcinogenic

Social media is an amazing tool for connecting, networking, building platforms, and entrepreneurship, and it provides a healthy dose of humor. I enjoy social media. Yet it feeds our natural human instinct to compare and is not a vehicle for intimacy. So many of our insecure thought patterns drive us toward comparison and isolation, and nothing feeds the cancer of comparison like the rogue thumbs we allow to scroll through everyone else's highlight reel on social media.

Comparison works for so many areas of our lives. For instance, if you're buying a new car, comparison is key, and chances are your real estate agent took you to more than one home because you needed to compare your options. And when choosing your wardrobe or a restaurant or a new flat-screen television, you should play the comparison game. But comparison is helpful only when options are present. The key word here is *options*.

But comparison doesn't help when it comes to decisions we've already made. Comparison isn't helpful when a man compares his wife to someone else's wife, because his wife isn't optional. She's a human being and represents a permanent decision he made before a community of people and God. And a woman's comparing her children to someone else's children is an act of futility, because her children are not optional. She can't swap them out for new, updated and upgraded versions.

Likewise, comparing your looks or your body to someone else's is pointless, because no options are available. You can scroll through every single photo that person you admire has ever posted, but nothing on their timeline is for sale, and despite how much you compare, you can never choose to have their life.

Comparison creates resentment toward our own choices and causes us to covet another person's life. Thoughts of comparison only drive us toward isolation and the Mind of Adam. Comparison is only a tool when it empowers us to make choices, not when it produces resentment toward self or jealousy toward others.

When we compare ourselves to others, we become isolated because it's quite difficult to build a healthy friendship with someone you've been secretly comparing yourself to. Also, comparison creates isolation, because if the object of our comparison isn't someone we have a real relationship with, we subconsciously devalue all the real people in our lives we've been comparing ourselves to.

Whenever I compare my reality to someone's fantasy life, I'll never come out of that exchange a winner. People don't post their real lives on social media. It's a curated platform, and the quickest way for me to be attacked with thoughts of discouragement, doubt, and defeat is to compare my messy reality with someone's perfected online persona.

Recently, I was at an event where someone approached me and said they were really excited to meet me. That made me excited to meet them. We were having a great conversation, and then they made a statement that made me nervous: "It's so cool to finally meet you in person, because it feels like I know you based on your Instagram." Immediately, I realized that our generation actually believes that what happens on Instagram is real. Although everything on my Instagram account is accurate, authentic, and honest, it isn't the entire truth. It wouldn't be possible nor wise to share my entire truth with the whole world. Maturity understands that a healthy lifestyle is based around concentric circles of relationship, and Jesus models this so well.

Jesus preached to crowds of hundreds and thousands.

Jesus traveled with His crew of twelve.

Jesus related to His core group of three.

Jesus revealed Himself to His closest friend.

Jesus had different circles, and each layer got a more intimate glance at the second Adam.

Jesus wasn't equipped or able to swim in the deep waters of relationship with hundreds of people, and I don't think we are either. But that doesn't stop us from trying. And we wonder why we're mentally exhausted, overwhelmed, stressed, and anxious? Instagram is for entertainment, not intimacy, and the more we try to use it for intimacy, the more frustrating life becomes. The goal is to cultivate deep relationships with a few people, but we've adopted this societal and generational pressure to be deep with everyone, which results in our feeling empty and drained.

Thoughts of comparison must be evicted if you're going to fully adopt the Mind of Christ and walk in mental freedom.

The Body of Christ

Could it be that the more individualistic and isolated our society becomes, the more vulnerable we become to forces like anxiety? As we keep our AirPods in to ignore the outside world, are we forfeiting our collective power to breathe in peace and exhale worry? Brain washing never happens in isolation, but it's always a social phenomenon as entire communities and cultures begin to march to the beat of the same drum. Could it be that we're so afraid of conforming to others that we've built walls that have locked us into our own private prison cells?

My fear is that many of us have tried to adopt the Mind of Christ without loving the body of Christ. Yes, the Mind of Christ is full of peace, full of joy, and full of identity, but we don't serve a decapitated Messiah. The beautifully flawed church is indeed the body and bride of Christ. We have no shortage of preaching via podcasts and sermons on YouTube, and we even livestream our "home church" services from the comfort of our homes.

But we're more lonely and isolated than ever. We've attempted to be connected to the Mind of Christ while amputated from the body of Christ. Could it be that the mind and body of Christ are irrevocably connected and that we will never receive the blessing of our Messiah's mind until we bear the burden of our Messiah's body?

I pray that we take all the tools Christ has equipped us with as we adopt the Mind of Christ and find our place in the body of Christ. Some may try to connect with His body and not His mind, or vice versa, but they're a package deal. The Mind of Christ is most available when we have deeply loved the universal body of Christ in godly community.

• • •

The Introduction to this book outlined our topic.

The next four chapters revealed the mess Adam got us into.

The middle two chapters showed us how Jesus got us out.

The following three chapters are the most practical part of this book. They're about thought patterns that can help us overcome anxiety, fear, doubt, harmful memories, and other types of toxic thoughts.

Let's move ahead.

PART THREE

Mind Maintenance

7

The Path to Peace

One day Jesus said to his disciples, "Let us go over to the other side of the lake." So they got into a boat and set out. As they sailed, he fell asleep. A squall came down on the lake, so that the boat was being swamped, and they were in great danger.

The disciples went and woke him, saying, "Master, Master, we're going to drown!" He got up and rebuked the wind and the raging waters; the storm subsided, and all was calm. "Where is your faith?" he asked his disciples.

In fear and amazement they asked one another, "Who is this? He commands even the winds and the water, and they obey him."

Luke 8:22–25

ANXIETY—THE OPPOSITE OF PEACE—is a cultural giant for our generation, and I have found two extreme responses to it in my pastoral journey. Neither approach seems to be working.

The first response is to condemn anxiety as sinful. I've heard many pastors remind people that Jesus commands His disciples to not be anxious. This approach leaves those of us who struggle with anxiety to feel ashamed and to hide the truth of our mental thought patterns. Inevitably, this strategy doesn't work, because shame and guilt can't produce the fruit of peace.

The second response is equally flawed and dangerous. Like a hospice nurse making dying patients comfortable during their last days, many pastors simply give people tools to cope with their anxious thoughts. When we passively accept our anxious thoughts and tendencies, we wave the white flag of surrender instead of fighting against anxiety. Much like Adam and Eve, when we fail to take a stand against anxiety, we don't die immediately. Yet surrendering to anxiety is a slow death. Jesus promised an abundant and full life to His followers, and anxiety doesn't fit the description of abundance and isn't compatible with the Mind of Christ.

As I said before, there's a ditch on either side of this narrow road crossing the bridge to the Mind of Christ, and therefore there's a ditch on either side on the path to peace. We try our best to avoid the ditch of condemnation as well as the ditch of coping and comfort. The disciple named John declared that Jesus was full of grace and truth (John 1:14) and that He didn't sacrifice either on the altar of the other. My prayer is that the Holy Spirit will help us balance grace and truth as we deal with this delicate topic. My prayer is that the same peace that governed the Mind of Christ while He slept through a storm on a boat will flood your mind as you read this chapter.

Let's jump in.

Nobody Ignores Turbulence Better Than . . .

My backpack was full of old boarding passes, and I had three flights coming up within the next week. But I found myself dreading the idea of boarding another plane.

Days passed, and my flight-triggered anxiety hadn't dissipated, so I nervously paced around the area at my departure gate, praying that the flight would be smooth and free of turbulence. Certainly,

Jesus had the power to keep the plane from experiencing turbulence, and I was confident that He loved me enough to honor my humble request—to intervene on the laws of aerodynamics and dispatch angels to hold the aircraft in such a way that there would be no turbulence. My intolerance for it was utterly incompatible with my airborne lifestyle and God's calling on my life, so either Jesus was going to answer my heartfelt and faith-filled prayers, or I would have to come up with a way to conquer my discomfort and panic.

If you're like me and turbulence brings immediate discomfort to your soul, then you'll be delighted to hear my praise report. God never answered that prayer. He did, however, perform an even greater miracle by giving me peace during my turbulent travel experience that day—and from then on.

Once we were in the air, the inevitable happened. We heard "unexpected rough air," the euphemism flight attendants use for the sake of the passengers on the brink of meltdown. I looked around and locked eyes with someone who seemed completely calm and unbothered. His peace wasn't immediately contagious—it was more of a slow burn—but by the end of that flight I had managed to relax more than usual, and I knew I was on to something.

Initially, I was amazed at how two people could encounter identical circumstances yet respond so differently. After looking into the nonchalant faces of several middle-aged businessmen, I was convinced that either something was wrong with my seat or they didn't care about their lives.

Eventually, staring into the stoic faces of fellow travelers became less of an indictment on them and more of an indictment on me. I was forced to conclude that since other people encountering the same scenario weren't scared, my fear was illogical. I stopped reacting to turbulence, and now I can sleep right through it. What I learned through my technique is that fear and peace are both deeply communal and contagious.

God doesn't stop turbulence; He uses it to grow our capacity for the chaos that surrounds us. And He gives us peace that surpasses all understanding. Jesus never promised us a trouble-free life. He does, however, have the power to create within us an anxiety-free life. The ultimate goal is to walk through trouble without being troubled by it. Our goal is to rest within a raging storm like Jesus did on a boat one day. If God had answered any of my original prayers, I would still be a slave to fear, and I would have forfeited a chance at authentic freedom.

I've observed many fearful and panicking travelers looking around and locking eyes with others. They begin their nonverbal communication with universal facial signals for panic and discomfort, and then fear begins to gain power over those others because panic is contagious.

Recently, I could sense the nervous tension of a man sitting next to me as we hit turbulence. I remembered being on edge and hypervigilant while flying, so I removed my AirPods and started talking to him. I watched this stranger's eyes as my peace began to have an effect on him because peace is equally contagious.

Years ago, I was flying to Boston from London when the plane decided to turn into a roller coaster. Just imagine several hundred life-sized bobblehead dolls riding across a cobblestone highway, and you'll begin to grasp what this flight felt like.

Nobody can ignore turbulence like a flight attendant, so to conquer my fear, I located the closest one with my eyes, and as long as she was calm, I convinced myself I was safe. As the turbulence got worse, though, her eyes closed, and she appeared to be praying. My suspicion was confirmed when she formed the sign of the crucifix from her forehead to her torso and then from one shoulder to the other. Panic filled the aircraft, because if the flight attendant, who must have known something the passengers didn't know, was scared, then logic would contend that we should all be scared too.

Panic in a Storm

In the same way turbulence must be abnormally strong for a flight attendant to be visibly afraid, a storm on the sea must be abnormally terrifying to have such an adverse effect on a group of men who have spent the majority of their lives on boats. The eighth chapter of Luke's Gospel describes a hectic scene where trained fishermen are crying out in despair as their lives flash before their eyes.

The scene starts with Jesus telling His disciples that they're headed to the other side of the lake, so the crew loads onto a boat and starts sailing toward the intended destination. Jesus falls asleep along the way, and then everything takes a turn for the worse. The Bible says a severe storm descends on the lake, and the disciples are certain they're going to die. The grip of fear tightens around the ship as these men reassure one another of their impending disaster. Jesus misses the initial mayhem of panic, but the disciples bring His nap to an abrupt end and demand that He do something about the storm.

In classic Christlike fashion, Jesus wakes up fully composed, because nobody can ignore turbulence like a flight attendant. Jesus speaks directly to the wind and the waves, commanding them to be calm, and then He addresses His scared disciples and asks them one of the most compelling questions in the entire New Testament. That question, recorded in Luke 8:25, changed the way I think about anxiety, fear, and worry.

The disciples are certain of what the wind and waves have the ability to do, and they've completely forgotten Jesus's words before they set sail. So after Jesus calms the storm, He hits them with this brick of a question: "Where is your faith?"

If someone asks, "Where is your car?" it means you have a car.

If someone asks, "Where is your spouse?" it means you have a spouse.

If someone asks, "Where is your pet llama?" it means you're Uncle Rico from the movie *Napoleon Dynamite* and I can't help you.

Logic follows that if someone asks, "Where is your faith?" it means you have faith. Jesus is not attacking their faith, but affirming and acknowledging the presence of their faith while simultaneously questioning and challenging the placement of their faith. If we carefully unpack Luke's account of this story, we'll discover the Mind of Christ on full display and the secret of taking our thoughts captive and unlocking lasting peace for the unexpectant turbulence of life and the raging storm within our souls. Jesus's question, "Where is your faith?" is not a command to discover faith they never had but a challenge to recover the faith they'd misplaced.

So where was their faith?

The disciples believed in what the storm had the power to do. They were certain it would kill them, and they imagined dying at its hand. They made a prediction based on the power they believed the storm possessed. They were convinced that the wind and the waves would overtake their boat and claim their lives.

Belief, certainty concerning the future, imagination, conviction, and prediction all sure do sound like the raw ingredients of faith to me.

The disciples were convinced of their impending doom.

The disciples imagined their own demise.

The disciples believed in their imminent destruction.

People with faith are convinced.

People with strong faith imagine.

People who live by faith believe.

I would contend that their faith was in the storm. I would contend that our faith is often found in the storm as well.

Jesus's question has little to do with the mediocrity or measurement of the disciples' faith but everything to do with the misplacement of their faith. Jesus typically provides feedback on the measurement of people's faith, but something radically more profound and helpful is happening in this event.

My goal is to help you flip over some couch cushions, search through some cupboards, empty out the trunk of your car, and find where you may have misplaced your faith. There's no need to feel guilty or condemned for not "having enough faith," because I'm certain that you currently have more faith than you're aware of.

In the same way that my keys being misplaced under the couch cushion prohibits my ability to operate my vehicle, when my faith is misplaced, my spiritual growth becomes stagnant and immobile. The Mind of Christ is full of faith, and operating the machinery of our minds properly requires the fuel of belief and imagination. Adopting the Mind of Christ requires that we locate all of our misplaced faith and fuel the engine of our minds properly.

To prove that you have more faith than you currently give yourself credit for, we're going to redefine worry, anxiety, and fear.

What is worry?

Worry is the ability to concentrate and meditate on a problem without ceasing. Worry requires focus, attention, meditation, imagination, and high mental capacity. Worrying is actually impressive.

I've struggled with ADHD my entire life. But when I'm worried, my ADHD can't even distract me from the rotating set of thoughts my mind is fixated on. A rather bittersweet discovery, I realized that my ability to worry meant that I also possessed the ability to focus and meditate. So I became determined to throw out the bathwater of worry but keep the proverbial baby of focus and meditation.

What is anxiety?

Anxiety takes root when we imagine an outcome that has not yet happened. Many times, we believe in that imagined future so much that we pull it from the realm of the invisible to the visible. Anxiety is when we give the imagined thoughts of the future so much power that we're physically overwhelmed by them.

What is fear?

Fear is an active acknowledgment of our human insufficiency and belief in the force of something greater than we are. Fear is being convinced of how that force could affect our existence.

It's impossible to worry without concentrating and meditating.
It's impossible to be anxious without using your imagination.
It's impossible to be afraid without believing in something
    greater than yourself.

At the root of worry, anxiety, and fear are the raw ingredients for faith. If they have consumed your mind, then this revelation should bring you infinite amounts of hope and joy. The worry, anxiety, and doubt you've experienced can become the launching pad into your most faith-filled days. All is not lost, and you have the seeds necessary to plant peace and the raw materials to build faith.

My wife and I have led and loved middle school students as well as adults who are medicated for and terrorized by anxious thoughts. Imagination is a consistent element found in the stories of the people I've pastored, and a key ingredient of anxiety is a fixation concerning an unknown outcome and the imagination to create an infinite number of destructive possibilities. Very often, someone will describe an event they're anxious over, but the event has not yet happened, the doomed scenarios are imaginary, and the threat lives in the realm of perception as opposed to reality.

Although the disciples were in a real storm, they imagined an outcome that did not come to pass. They imagined that they would drown, and they had proof and good reason for that deduction. But they were still wrong. Just because proof and good reason to doubt exist doesn't excuse misplaced faith.

Do you know what typically happens when you use your mind's creativity and imaginative power to fixate on something that has yet to occur? For starters, whatever it is typically occurs. Because where you direct your creativity and imagination is the place where your faith can be found, and faith brings those things that don't yet exist into the realm of reality. Faith doesn't discriminate between good and bad or unhealthy and functional. Faith can usher healing from the unseen realm into reality, and faith can also bring sickness from the unseen realm into reality.

Faith is a powerful weapon that can be used to sabotage your future or to create the abundant life Jesus promised. Faith works equally for our breakthrough as well as our breakdown. If the power of your imagination has been at work pulling failure from the future into your present, then through Christ you can use that same imagination to begin creating God's ideal future for your life.

Jesus woke up and immediately sensed the power of faith at work on the boat. But the disciples' faith was not working for them but against them. The placement of their faith was killing them, and they learned that their faith was better off placed in a sleeping Messiah than in the eye of a raging storm.

If you have ever felt swept away under the powerful currents of negative thoughts, drowning under the weight of worry or caught in the undertow of unbelief, I promise you that Jesus has the power to rescue your anxious heart and renew your troubled mind. In the Gospels we observe the Mind of Christ in action through the words, actions, and teachings of Jesus. Jesus walks with His disciples as they slowly abandon the Mind of Adam and adopt Jesus's way of thinking, and Luke gives us a glimpse into this process as they're all aboard a nearly shipwrecked sea vessel.

The storm found in Luke's Gospel is a necessary stop on the journey from the Mind of Adam to the Mind of Christ so that we can also learn how to harness and redirect negative mental energy. The Mind of Christ gives every believer the power and authority to transform their negative thought patterns. Like water being turned into wine, our worry, anxiety, and fear can be transformed into the powerful currents of peace and faith we need. The Mind of Christ harnesses the power of anxiety, using it to our advantage.

Harnessing Our Humanity

If you've ever visited Niagara Falls, you've seen the transformative power of renewed thinking at work. The water roars like thunder as it collapses at the bottom of the 165-foot drop, and beneath your feet you can feel the vibrating force of nature's subwoofer. The sheer power of the falls is inescapable, and although there's safety from the observation deck, it's clear that nobody would survive Niagara Falls if they were to dare venture beyond the safety of the guardrails. With more than six million cubic feet of water going over the crest of the falls every minute, Niagara Falls is undeniably the most powerful waterfall in North America, and the overwhelming and unfiltered power of nature is on display as you approach.

The falls have claimed a long list of lives, including daredevils and stuntmen who never lived to tell about their experiences. Yet despite all the danger associated with this powerful force of nature, the power of Niagara Falls is constantly being harnessed for the benefit of humanity in the form of hydroelectricity. The hydroelectric plants along the Niagara River provide power for hundreds of thousands of homes.

Harnessing hydroelectric power proves that although something has the power to destroy humanity, it may have the power to develop humanity as well. The same force of power that can destroy one person's life also has the ability to bring necessary development to entire communities of people. Whether the river is being used for destruction or harnessed for the destiny and development of humanity is a matter of our decisions.

When Adam and Eve ate from the forbidden tree, the will of humanity was placed under the debilitating control of sin, and under the Mind of Adam our decision-making skills have been severely impaired. The Mind of Adam is in a perpetual state of intoxicated stupor, but the Mind of Christ lifts our minds out of the fog and gives us the power to make wise decisions. Under the Mind of Christ, we can decide to harness the power of anxiety and fear and transform them into the fuel necessary for the engine of faith to operate.

Anxiety and Control

My first therapist taught me a phrase years ago, and the moment he said the words, I could feel the stronghold of control melt and lose its power. He said, "The best control is self-control." He then had me write down everything I currently had control over in my life. This seemed like a silly activity, but every time I declared I was done he would make me continue. By the end of the session, I had a massive list of things I had control over.

The Serpent's trick is to make us forfeit the things under our control by showing us all the things we can't control. When the storms of life start raging out of control, he tells us we've lost control of everything in our lives. Nothing could be further from the truth. The moment we begin to believe his lie—that we've lost control of our lives—is when we feel overwhelmed and anxiety gains a foothold in our souls.

Perhaps you need to stop reading right now and remind yourself of everything you have control over versus what you don't.

You don't have control over . . .

- the past or future.
- other people.
- God.

- your spouse.
- the turbulence.

But you do have control over . . .
- your mood.
- your decisions.
- your time.
- your present moments.
- your words.
- your passion.
- your emotions.
- your will.
- your fight.
- your resilience.
- your determination.
- your pride.
- your gifts.
- your talents.
- your unique genius.
- your empathy.
- your weaknesses.
- your strengths.
- your response to turbulence.
- your thoughts.

When you compare lists, you realize that the number of things you can control is infinitely more impressive than the number of things you can't control.

The Serpent enjoys baiting us with the allure of control over what we can't control, but every time we take the bait, we end up with less of what we wanted in the first place. Our foreparents fell prey to the same deceitful tactic. They wanted to be like God, knowing good and evil, and they placed the very image of God they possessed in jeopardy. They lost their control by chasing more control, and the children of Adam and Eve have been cursed with the chaotic chase for control ever since. At the end of the chase, the only thing we catch is our anxious souls. The Serpent appears within the winds and waves of life to convince us that we have no control over our lives. But as long as you have control over yourself and your soul, you can always tame the sea and the storm.

Jesus woke up and had the authority to calm the storm because He had already calmed His own soul. He had authority and control over His mind, His will, and His emotions, and so He also had authority over the storm.

Authority flows outward, so we'll never have authority over the storms around us until we first gain control over the storms within us. It's exponentially more difficult to tame the storms of life than it is to tame the storms within our souls. Dominion over self, however, always leads to dominion over storms. Remember, only when Adam lost dominion over himself did everything within creation cease to obey him. Jesus reverses the rebellion of creation by regaining authority over Himself through the submitted will evident in the garden of Gethsemane. In one garden humanity lost control. In another garden humanity regained control by returning the crown to its rightful owner.

Lucifer Still Wants Worship

How can we be so sure that the disciples' faith was misplaced in the storm? Because Satan has proven that there's one thing he desires above all else: worship.

Lucifer's eviction from heaven was due to his desire to receive glory instead of reflect God's glory. The archangel desired worship above all else and pushed all his chips to the center of the table and took the gamble of eternity. His lust for worship continued into the New Testament when he tried to deceive Jesus into exchanging a couple of moments of worship for the kingdoms of the earth. The biblical evidence is stacked against the old angel of light, and it's clear that this father of lies desires worship more than anything else. Yet when we think of Satan worship, we typically think of images from *The Exorcist*, heavy metal, gothic clothing, animal sacrifices, mediums, witches, warlocks, inverted pentagrams, and all things Wiccan.

But what if Satan is smarter than that?

What if he wraps himself in the winds and waves of life?

I don't know how many converts Satan would win if worshiping him required that his followers unbox their nearest Ouija board and tattoo an inverted pentagram on their foreheads, but if he were crafty, he'd deceive humans into misplacing our faith until it was securely rooted within the storms of life. If we're not careful, we'll find ourselves consumed with how the Serpent is attacking us, and it will be the only thing we talk about.

I refuse to be impressed with how the Serpent is opposing me, and I refuse to give him any free publicity.

Enough Said

The apostle Paul is clear that "faith comes by hearing, and hearing by the word of God" (Romans 10:17 NKJV). So our faith should always be in the word that God has spoken as opposed to the storm we see. Like the disciples, we often have more faith in the storms surrounding us than in the word that is sustaining us. Before Jesus fell asleep on the boat, He spoke to the disciples, and their faith should have been firmly planted in His words: "Let us go over to the other side of the lake" (Luke 8:22).

Once Jesus gave the disciples a definitive plan for the destination of the vessel, no storm could stop them. The storm in the middle of the journey is simply a distraction from the words Jesus spoke concerning their destination. The moment a storm begins to break out and fights for my mental allegiance, I must remember that my destination has been predetermined. Jesus is the author and finisher of my faith, and He's declared that He and I are going to the other side of the lake.

Once we place our faith, trust, and unwavering conviction in the words God has spoken, we begin to laugh at storms. This is why Jesus had the ability to take a nap in the middle of apparent danger. The secret of peace is to focus on the promised destination instead of the threatening distraction. If we're going to win the battle against fear, worry, and anxiety, we must have more faith in the words of the rabbi who's sleeping in the bottom of our boat than we have in the storm. We must believe that God is faithful and that like the author of Numbers declares, "God is not human, that he should lie; not a human being, that he should change his mind" (23:19).

And we must agree with the prophet Isaiah, who was adamant that "as the rain and the snow come down from heaven, and do not return to it without watering the earth and making it bud and flourish . . . so is my word that goes out from my mouth: It will not return to me empty, but will accomplish what I desire and achieve the purpose for which I sent it" (Isaiah 55:10–11).

God isn't keen on giving lots of details or vast colorful explanations. So the irony of faith is that the location that seems the riskiest is the only secure place for our faith to rest. Faith seems foolish according to secular logic, but the life of Noah proves that on the day of the storm, the faithful will be vindicated for trusting in the word God has spoken.

Even before Tia and I got married, God prompted separate random people to tell her she would be an amazing mother one day. On multiple occasions people walked up to her and said things like, "I saw you holding children, and they were yours." At the time it seemed not only random but out of place. Not only was Tia single, but she was also a virgin. So to say the least, receiving prophetic words about children was slightly stressful. God has been known to impregnate a virgin, but Tia wanted no part of that miracle.

Eventually, we got married, and deciding it was time to fill the world with more Arangos, we began trying. After the first couple of months of failing to conceive, however, we were both panicking and afraid to admit it to each other. Then the ice shattered, and the months of disappointment flooded the conversation. An entire year of trying to get pregnant passed before we visited the fertility clinic for the first time, and we'll never forget how the doctor's diagnosis sounded more like a judge's verdict. It felt like we'd been sentenced to a life of barrenness.

As we sat in our car decompressing, I remembered all those random people approaching Tia years prior to tell her she'd be an amazing mom. We began to see those random words as deliberate promises from a loving God.

In the middle of this infertility storm, God's promise over us was the anchor to our faith. We'd already been on a journey of infertility for years, with a lot of turbulence. But our faith was not in medicine, doctors, money, or any of the diagnoses we'd received. I believe in the promises of God more than any storm the Serpent has the power to wrap himself in.

The nurses and doctors at our clinic loved us because we brought joy into a relatively sad environment. The source of our joy wasn't in our health or the possibility of having children. The source of our peace wasn't in the finances necessary for expensive fertility treatment. The source of our peace was in something that can never be taken away, and I'm convinced that when we Christians decide to place our faith in the unshakable foundation of God's loving promises, our peace will become a magnetic draw to a world filled with anxiety. The church doesn't need more trendy marketing campaigns. It needs to place the supply of our unshakable peace on display because there is currently a record-high demand for peace.

Tia and I prayed together, cried together, and encouraged each other. And every single month we believed for good news. Yet for so long we were disappointed. Still, we'd rather believe God and be disappointed than believe in the storm and drown in the sea of nonchalance.

The disciples didn't realize that when Jesus said, "Let us go over to the other side of the lake" He was giving them a promise to stand on. And Tia didn't realize that God was giving her a promise when random people spoke to her concerning her future.

So what promises has the Lord given you? Before the storm. Before the nap. What did He say?

Did He say you would get through the divorce?

Did He say your entire family would be born again?

Did He say you would be healed?

Did He say you could overcome the addiction?

Did He say you would walk in forgiveness?

There's almost always a disconnect between what God has spoken and what we see in front of us, but faith makes up the difference in that gap. Faith is what closes the gap between His promise and our present. Faith is the anchor that keeps anxiety and fear from capsizing our boat.

So where is your faith?

Don't Feed the Monkeys

To be loved but not known is comforting but superficial. To be known and not loved is our greatest fear. But to be fully known and truly loved is, well, a lot like being loved by God. It is what we need more than anything. It liberates us from pretense, humbles us out of our self-righteousness, and fortifies us for any difficulty life can throw at us.

Timothy Keller[1]

The rabble with them began to crave other food, and again the Israelites started wailing and said, "If only we had meat to eat! We remember the fish we ate in Egypt at no cost—also the cucumbers, melons, leeks, onions and garlic. But now we have lost our appetite; we never see anything but this manna!"

Numbers 11:4–6

MY HEART SEEMED TO DROP into my stomach when my wife held up my recent Instagram search history and asked why I'd been visiting my ex-girlfriend's profile on my phone. I was stunned, speechless—and inwardly scheming a way to get myself out of this predicament. I was both naked and very ashamed. Even though she'd caught me, I still wanted to grasp for a cover-up, an excuse, a defense, anything.

Tia and I had been married for only a few months, and I could see the honeymoon phase crashing and burning in her eyes. I was scared she'd be angry. I was scared that her feelings would be hurt. Ultimately, I was scared of losing the intimacy while it was still in its infancy, and when we're scared, we cover up, we become defensive, and we hide.

Hours later I learned that perfect love does cast out all fear, because that was no longer a cliche from a Bible verse but an experience I walked through in my heart. At some point during this uncomfortable conversation, I realized that although my wife was indeed hurt—and disappointed—she wasn't going anywhere, and I could let down my guard, take off my fig leaves, and be honest.

I was afraid of losing intimacy with a woman I loved more than anyone, so I hid. But then I was shocked, because by the end of the conversation my deepest fears hadn't come true. It's so ironic that as I began to come clean, my honesty built intimacy instead of tearing it down. I'm glad that my wife wouldn't accept easy answers from me. I'm glad she confronted me. I'm glad she kept pressing when I gave surface-level answers, because I needed an explanation for my actions even more than she did. Although I'd known what I was doing, I wasn't aware of why I was doing it or how it was damaging my thought life.

Genesis records that the first human couple "knew" each other, and that the woman conceived and gave birth to a son (Genesis 4:1 NKJV). The Bible describes marriage and sexual intimacy as a deep knowledge, as if both parties have studied each other. It describes a process whereby lovers dissect and decipher each other in detailed adoration and respect. The intimacy of love fuels infatuation as well as inspection as they search the depths of each other's soul.

This is the scariest part of marriage. There's a risk attached to being fully known, and it's the fear of rejection. As Timothy Keller says in his book *The Meaning of Marriage*, "To be known and not loved is our greatest fear."[2] That's a brilliant way to echo God's heart when He says that "perfect love casts out fear" (1 John 4:18 NKJV). When we're loved by God and loved well by others, there is no fear of rejection.

Thanks to the Mind of Adam, my wife's inspection felt like interrogation to me because of my own guilt and pride. Her question hit me like I was being sucker punched—the initial shock of being deeply and fully known. Once I entered into a marital covenant, I inaugurated a constant state of being known by someone and knowing them as well. I was "naked," but whether I'd be ashamed was in my control. Unfortunately, some married couples can't handle the depth of intimacy, and so they hide and keep secrets. But in doing so, they rob their marriage of a powerful gift.

Many of us rob ourselves of the same gift when it comes to our relationship with God. We avoid His light, which exposes every area of our lives. We keep Him an arm's length away. We hide. We cover up. And then we're disappointed when the relationship doesn't yield the results we'd hoped for.

As we've seen in John 15:4–5, Jesus told His disciples that if they remained in Him and His words remained in them, they would bear much fruit. This sounds incredibly similar to the relationship between the first two humans. Again, Genesis 4:1 tells us Adam "knew" his wife, Eve, and that she conceived and had a son. The Bible seems to teach that intimate knowledge is the only path to fruitfulness and that isolation always results in barrenness. In the same way some people have a shallow or empty marriage because they fear full disclosure, some of us have a shallow, empty, and unfruitful relationship with God for the same reason. We're either going to be laid bare before God or barren before God. The choice is between being uncovered or unfruitful. The truth is that fruitfulness requires full disclosure.

For weeks leading up to my wife's fateful confrontation, I'd stumbled across or even searched for my ex-girlfriend's Instagram page. And each time I found it, I also found myself further and further toward the bottom of her account. Quick glances had started turning into full-blown recaps and replays as I relived moments we'd had together in my mind.

The first time this happened it was innocent; someone tagged her in a photo, and I spent a couple of seconds on her page. But eventually what began as innocent became intentional, and I was slowly enticed to explore and enjoy the playground of my memories. Each photo was like a new ride, and it's not long before memories become romanticized and exaggerated. Once I felt safe to be honest and turned my wife's inspection into introspection, I came to a realization that has changed my life, and I pray it will change yours.

I told Tia that looking at this ex-girlfriend's Instagram made me realize I missed some things about that relationship. But she had been around to observe the relationship I was describing, and she reminded me of how toxic that relationship had been and how unhappy I'd been. She reminded me of how emotionally manipulative it was and how everyone around me and this other young lady talked about the toxicity of the relationship. My wife reminded me of the truth because my memories weren't able to.

This may come as a surprise to you, but our memories simply aren't trustworthy, accurate, or helpful. Nothing will damage the life of your mind more than giving power to memories that replay half-truths. We can't spend time in the playground of memories and expect to be clear-minded, mentally sharp, or wise when we choose to snap out of it and reenter the real world. Memories have a gravitational pull, and it takes discipline and accountability to escape their orbit. Nothing will infect the mind of the believer as quickly as the destructive power of a toxic memory. Memories easily get turned into fantasies and will ultimately turn reality into a nightmare.

By feeding my memories, I was forcing my wife to compete with an inaccurate and exaggerated version of my past, and she was doomed to lose this imaginary competition every time.

The truth is I'm not alone in this. Many of us have trouble breaking free of the maze of memories we've wandered into. We tell ourselves we won't wander too far, but eventually, we all lose track of time in the maze of memories. And then before we're aware of it, we don't know how to get out. My memories of the past almost kept me from appreciating the miracle of being married to Tia.

The Miracle of Manna

Even if you don't know it from reading the Bible, if you've ever seen *The Ten Commandments* starring Charlton Heston or *The Prince of Egypt*, you should be familiar with the story of Moses, Pharaoh, and the enslaved people of Israel. For hundreds of years the people of Israel lived under harsh captivity as slaves in Egypt. At one point the Egyptians even killed all the male Israelite children under the age of two. Life for God's people was full of mental oppression, hard labor, physical bondage, and emotional misery. They lived under the constant threat of punishment, torture, and death, which provoked them to cry out to God for deliverance.

Finally, after centuries of this harsh treatment, God answers the cry of their hearts, and through a series of miraculous events, their chains are broken. Their dreams come true, and their prayers are answered in radical fashion. God shows off His power and might during this epic portion of the Bible with plagues, pillars of fire, and His parting of the Red Sea. Seriously, if you've never seen *The Prince of Egypt*, you've been deprived.

The people are free from Egypt and head toward Canaan, the land God promised to give them to possess. But they must travel through the wilderness to get there, and they need food. They can't grow any crops because they're nomads and the land isn't fertile.

So God performs a miracle. Every single morning, the dew on the ground miraculously turns into bread they can collect and use to feed their households. The people refer to this miracle bread as manna, and every day God demonstrates His care and concern by providing this food for His people. That should be the end of the story, but unfortunately, the Israelites begin to complain.

In Numbers 11:4–6, the Bible describes how the people of Israel allow their memories to rob them of their miracle:

> The rabble with them began to crave other food, and again the Israelites started wailing and said, "If only we had meat to eat! We remember the fish we ate in Egypt at no cost—also the cucumbers, melons, leeks, onions and garlic. But now we have lost our appetite; we never see anything but this manna!"

I've found that whenever the seasons of life bring challenge, uncertainty, or stress, my memories are right there to comfort me and offer a momentary escape from reality. This happens to all of us, but we can't take the bait. The people of Israel reminisce about the "good ole days" when they had more certainty, more security, more predictability, more options on the menu.

The good ole days . . .
- more melons
- more leeks
- more cucumbers
- more fish

But also . . .
- chains
- whips
- abuse
- slavery

And for some of us?

The good ole days . . .

- gifts
- compliments
- romance
- chemistry

But also . . .

- arguments
- dysfunction
- stress
- insecurities

When we reminisce about and dwell on the past, we allow inaccurate information to camouflage as truth and taint our ability to discern God's will. We all need somebody to remind us that the good ole days weren't really as good as we remember them to be, and that nothing in the past is worth jeopardizing the miracle of the present moment God has brought us to.

I can empathize with the children of Israel. The journey through the wilderness isn't easy, and it's unpredictable. The season you're in right now may not be ideal; it may not be Canaan. But it's better than Egypt, and no matter the difficulty, it beats being enslaved.

Stop flirting with your past, let those flames completely die out, and march forward with tunnel vision toward the future God has mapped out for you.

All the sons and daughters of Adam have amnesia mixed with romantic nostalgia, which makes the playground of memories especially unsafe. Certain details get exaggerated. Certain uncomfortable details get suppressed. Some memories get conveniently omitted altogether. The jungle gym of journal entries and the slippery slide of sentimental keepsakes have an allure, but you're more likely to cause harm to your mind than you are to have fun. You're very likely to start swinging on the monkey bars of your memories and get injured on the rusty and dilapidated equipment. Memory Lane has killer potholes that can derail your judgment and trigger confusion, indecisiveness, unnecessary regret, and overall mental turmoil. The Serpent knows about this malfunction and masterfully manipulates our memories, trying to sabotage God's plan for our lives.

The journey from Egypt to Canaan could not be made without traveling through the transitional terrain of the wilderness. Canaan is where the Israelites would settle. Egypt was where they were slaves. The wilderness was only a season. Seasons of transition are marked with stressful uncertainty, and the land of familiarity is still in earshot and promises that you can return at no cost. The secret to this season is to starve all memories of the past and keep moving toward Canaan.

That night I learned a powerful lesson that I immediately put into practice. This lesson is simple, but I promise that when applied to your life, it will yield amazing results. Here it is:

Whatever you starve will die.

Whatever you feed will grow.

Memories are like plants that live in the soil of your mind. Every time you open the file and sift through the contents, you feed that memory. Every time you entertain flashbacks, you feed that memory. Sometimes we feed memories a consistent diet of our mental attention, and then we're shocked when they've become a stronghold in our thinking. Negative thoughts are like parasites that derive all their strength from the host with the intention of killing it one day. We nourish negative thoughts and help them grow so strong that eventually we aren't strong enough to overpower them.

Not until I stopped feeding the memories did they shrivel and wither away. That night I made a vow to my wife, to myself, and to God that I would no longer entertain memories of a season He rescued me from. So I deleted certain social media apps from my phone, I unfollowed certain people, and I removed all detour signs that would fight for my attention and ultimately distract me from my destiny. You can do the exact same thing and regain control of your mind.

The real key in this process isn't to think about how you need to take dominion over your mind, and it isn't to focus on expelling old memories. That's useful, but eventually you'll start thinking about the very thing you don't want to think about. The real key to finding contentment while in a season of transition is to focus your mind on everything God has rescued you from.

That's exactly what helped me. I stopped focusing on what I needed to do and started focusing on what God had already done. I started to worship God and hold His work in my life in higher esteem. I began to reflect and recount all the ways He delivered me from that toxic relationship. It's impossible to be thankful to God for deliverance and simultaneously fantasize about the season He's delivered you from.

Instead of thinking back on the meat, melons, and leeks, the Israelites could have easily remembered how the Nile turned to blood; how darkness, frogs, and locusts covered the land; how hail and fire rained down from heaven to break Pharaoh's grasp on them; and ultimately, how the Red Sea opened up to reveal a path of dry ground and then swallowed the Egyptian army. The people of Israel should have been sitting around the fire at night telling the story of how God miraculously delivered them with a mighty hand and an outstretched arm. While they ate their manna, they should have meditated on the miracle of their own deliverance.

Nothing helps us appreciate the miracles of the present season more than meditating on the miracles of the previous season.

Meditating on the miracle of your emancipation will cause your mind to appreciate and value the miracle of manna even when the Serpent wants to tempt you with memories of meat.

The Miracle of Rehab

My dad took me to a crack house when I was five years old. The reason that night is etched in my memory is that it was the night before my parents got married. My mom was definitely the responsible caregiver of our family, and I would have been with her that night. But her friends threw her a bachelorette party, so my dad and I had a "guys' night out."

His drug addiction turned my childhood into a roller coaster, where nothing was ever predictable.

Then after twenty-five years of marriage, my mom finally wanted to get off the ride. My pastor decided to mediate a conversation between my parents and wanted me present, and my mom expressed that she simply couldn't take the emotional turmoil and indirect abuse that came as a result of my father's addiction. Like countless times before, my dad promised to quit—cold turkey. He had his script prepared and memorized. But this time my mother had his script memorized as well, and she wasn't budging.

My pastor interrupted the stalemate with a radical idea. He suggested that my father participate in a Christian rehabilitation program for men, and he was even willing to pay for all the expenses related to it.

Dad asked three questions:

1. "Will I have to live in a dorm-style room with a bunk bed and an assigned roommate?"
2. "Is there a cafeteria where I'll have to eat whatever food is provided?"
3. "Is there a set time to wake up as well as a curfew?"

Each answer was yes, and right away I knew he wouldn't attend the program. Dad had spent eighteen years in prison while he was still living in Cuba, and he'd vowed to never return. I saw Manny Arango Sr.'s response coming like a Facebook ad right after I Google a new product. He looked at my pastor and said, "Man, that's prison. I'm not going there."

The Christian rehab program was a real chance at freedom, but Dad saw it as bondage. He couldn't see that the crack house he frequented was actually more prison-like. My father's mind was not capable of processing such a radical thought. Manny Arango Sr. couldn't accept the thought of an inpatient rehab program because he needed a new mind, not simply a new idea.

The timeless truth is that the Mind of Adam will always reject the thoughts of Christ. Our minds in their natural fallen state tend to distort reality, and like Adam, we call God's loving moral truth tyrannical and controlling. Especially when looking through the lens of our painful past experiences, we will constantly reject God's attempt to bring us into unfamiliar freedom. My dad refused to do anything that made him feel like an inmate and effectively forfeited his chance of ever escaping the imprisonment of addiction. Sadly, he confused moral independence with genuine freedom, and my fear is that many of us are rejecting new thoughts because we're utilizing old minds and mindsets. Again, my dad didn't simply need a new thought or idea; he needed a new mind. And although he had received Christ as his Savior, he never adopted the Mind of Christ that was available to him, and he remained stuck in bondage.

As I listened to Manny Arango Sr. compare rehab to prison, I was reminded of the Sistine Chapel. The disappointment I had in my dad may have sparked my mind to remember the hope to which the Christian faith is anchored. Just as Michelangelo depicted, God is still holding out His finger to humankind, willing to impart wisdom, understanding, and mental clarity. Adam may have gotten our species into a web of confusion, but Jesus offers every single believer a new mind.

The people of Israel couldn't appreciate the miracle of the manna because their minds were stuck on the memory of the old menu. The passage we studied from the book of Numbers is one of the most heartbreaking stories in the Bible. They were willing to forfeit everything God had promised just to regain what they perceived as a loss.

It's a lot like an addict who can't appreciate the miracle of rehab because his memory of prison colors his present opportunity.

It's a lot like a new husband who can't fully appreciate the beauty and favor of his bride because she's being compared to a distorted memory of the past.

I know my father and I aren't the only people who struggle with this. Which one of your memories is making your miracles seem mundane and mediocre?

Don't Feed the Monkeys

The first time I visited South Africa, I fell completely in love. The people are so kind and hospitable, and the culture and history of the nation are rich with diversity and stories of triumph. The team I was with explored the country for an entire month. We went on safari, and we even visited Nelson Mandela's former prison cell.

One of my lasting memories is having to fight monkeys for my lunch! Our whole squad had hiked up a mountain and decided to have lunch at the top, and I immediately noticed that the place was littered with signs that read Don't Feed the Monkeys! It quickly became evident that most people ignored the signs, because most people were feeding them, and monkeys were everywhere.

Whoever put up those signs knew best. Because people fed the monkeys, they came around expecting something to eat and aggressively snatched food from hikers. Feeding the monkeys led to expectation, and that expectation led to aggression. The sign was clear: Don't Feed the Monkeys! And when it comes to adopting the Mind of Christ, the sign is just as clear: Don't Feed the Memories! If you feed the harmful memories in your mind, they'll grow and become aggressive. But if you starve them, they'll die.

The Mind of Christ has the ability to remove memories when we meditate on the miraculous power of God. The Mind of Christ also has the power to redeem the painful memories that plague and torment believers, and we'll explore that next as we continue to travel from the Mind of Adam to the Mind of Christ.

9

Garden Snakes and Wooden Horses

When an impure spirit comes out of a person, it goes through arid places seeking rest and does not find it. Then it says, "I will return to the house I left." When it arrives, it finds the house unoccupied, swept clean and put in order. Then it goes and takes with it seven other spirits more wicked than itself, and they go in and live there. And the final condition of that person is worse than the first.

Matthew 12:43–45

Finally, brothers and sisters, whatever is true, whatever is noble, whatever is right, whatever is pure, whatever is lovely, whatever is admirable—if anything is excellent or praiseworthy—think about such things.

Philippians 4:8

Set your minds on things above, not on earthly things.

Colossians 3:2

Do not give the devil a foothold.

Ephesians 4:27

I RECKLESSLY RAN through our townhouse playing tag with my wife one day as if she were my grade school crush, trying to avoid being tickled. Tia darted up the stairs to seek asylum in our bedroom. Luckily, I got to the door milliseconds before she could shut it and managed to wedge my foot at its base. I was only inches away from Tia, but the door protected her ticklish rib cage from my hands.

The protection of the door, however, was far from permanent, thanks to the foothold I'd managed to achieve. Before long I was able to wiggle my knee into the crevice, and next I had an arm inside the bedroom. Tia put up a valiant defense, but the power of a single foothold can't be underestimated. I snuck my shoulder through next, followed by my hip, and then it was over. I was in.

This silly and lighthearted story demonstrates exactly how the Serpent creates mental strongholds in our minds. Strongholds always start as footholds. In Ephesians 4:27, Paul teaches the Ephesian church not to give Satan a foothold, because the moment we start to entertain the slightest of poisonous thoughts, the sand in the hourglass is set in motion. It won't be long before that thought begins to gain control of our thinking.

Unforgiveness can't be entertained.

Temptation can't be given an audience.

Insecurity must not be listened to.

We can't flirt with destructive thoughts.

A small foothold will indeed end with the Serpent in your room, establishing his stronghold in your mind.

Curiosity caused Adam and Eve to stand at the Tree of Knowledge with the Serpent and give audience and attention to hypnotizing half-truths. The strongholds of insecurity, abandonment, or pessimism can often be traced back to a small foothold that can become the key to our freedom. The Serpent will strategically sow seeds while we're young and defenseless, and then like a gardener, he works tirelessly to bring those seeds to maturity within our vulnerable minds.

Fortunately, the Mind of Adam begins to unravel like a cheap sweater when the foothold of our toxic thought patterns is identified. The Mind of Christ gives us the revelation necessary to identify the seed-like footholds and regain mental freedom. The Mind of Christ gives believers the power to piece together the fragments of our memories until we discover the genesis of a thought.

When I was six years old, my dad was scheduled to perform a routine pickup after school to take me home. I waved goodbye to most of my friends as their parents came on time, and then, with my father late, I took his tardiness as an opportunity to relive the glory of recess with my friends who remained.

But soon the crowd dwindled down to ten.

Then five.

Then one.

The concrete steps of St. Patrick's Elementary School in the Boston neighborhood of Roxbury were where I made friends with the police officer who waited with me until Dad showed up hours later. The Serpent saw his opportunity and exploited it.

More than thirty years have passed since that experience, yet it's permanently sketched on the chalkboard of my memory. That single memory became the garden where the Serpent worked diligently to create a mental stronghold of abandonment, insecurity, mistrust, and unforgiveness.

Years ago, I desperately wanted to be free from the web of thoughts that entangled me, and just like the Holy Spirit drove Jesus into the wilderness, I was forced to walk up those concrete steps of St. Patrick's and dig up seeds the Serpent had planted in the mind of a scared first-grade boy.

As I looked up the stairs, the Holy Spirit began to show me that He'd sent that police officer to protect me. The Spirit of God had formed a hedge of protection around me, ensuring that I wouldn't be kidnapped or abused. My heavenly Father began to reveal that, as He did with young Samuel, He was training my ear to hear His voice and sense His presence at a young age. The Mind of Christ began to show me that although I was hard-pressed on every side, I was not crushed that day. I was certainly perplexed, but I was not in despair on those concrete steps. I was persecuted by the Serpent but not abandoned by God. I was struck down by a foothold but not destroyed by a stronghold.

The Mind of Christ revealed the origin of a mental stronghold, and then it gave me new perspective on a memory that had previously haunted me. The Mind of Christ redeemed that memory so that now I can look back and, like David, declare that "though my father and mother forsake me, the LORD will receive me" (Psalm 27:10). The Mind of Christ reversed the stronghold and loosened the grip of Satan's influence over my thinking. The Mind of Adam is powerless to crush the Serpent, but hidden within the aftermath of Adam and Eve's failure is a promise that a Messiah will rise and prove victorious over every seed-watering lie that slips from the Serpent's slithering tongue.

Defensive Playbook

Childhood isn't the only season of our lives when the Serpent has an open door to plant seeds of destruction in the soil of our minds. Satan and his minions are busy conniving their way into the lives of adults, too, and if like me you've seen the movie *Troy*, then you've seen another one of hell's deceitful tactics at work.

As I recall from both school and that film, the Greeks had fruitlessly laid siege to the city of Troy for ten long years. Ancient cities like Troy were protected and defended by intimidatingly fortified walls, which left an opposing army with a handful of options. When faced with the impenetrable walls of a well-fortified city, some armies still attempted an attack by scaling the walls with ladders and siege ramps that resembled scaffolding. That, however, wasn't always successful. It's exponentially more difficult to climb a wall and overthrow a city than it is for soldiers to take their post at the top of the wall and shoot arrows down at their enemy targets—or worse, to pour boiling hot lead and other molten metals on the heads of enemy climbers.

The next option for overtaking a walled city was to use a battering ram on the gates of the city. Whereas the walls were made of stone, the gates were often made of wood and therefore were the most vulnerable parts of the wall. The gates had to be made of wood in order to allow citizens to freely enter and exit their city.

The final option was to allow the impenetrable city to become a prison for the inhabitants, cutting them off from food, water, and other basic human needs. During a siege the gates of the city would be permanently locked and sealed for protection, but once the city ran out of food, that protection became a prison. Armies would simply wait until the citizens of the city resorted to cannibalism and then eventually surrendered.

None of these proven tactics worked for the Greeks, and ten fruitless years passed as the city of Troy seemed unbothered by the surrounding siege.

The Greeks had sailed all the way to Troy, encamped around their city, sacrificed the blood of their soldiers and a decade of their lives only to find that their army was no match for the walls of Troy. But they couldn't bear the thought of accepting defeat, so they took a page from the Serpent's playbook and devised a rather crafty plan to overthrow the Trojans.

They constructed a massive and hollow horse made of wood, later known as the Trojan Horse. Then they filled it with soldiers and pretended to sail away, leaving behind this parting gift for their "victorious" opponents. The Trojans pulled the horse into their city, and that night the hidden soldiers crept out of the horse and opened the gates for the rest of the Greek army, which had sailed back under cover of night. The Greeks entered and destroyed the city of Troy, ending the war.

Paul teaches the Philippian church that, like a walled city, our minds are protected against the Serpent as we adopt the Mind of Christ. As the peace of Christ guards our minds, the Serpent is left with only a handful of options for how to attack us. Like an enemy army attacking the gates of a city, the Serpent rigorously attacks our access points. The most vulnerable gates to the human mind are the ears and eyes, and Satan sleeplessly works to invade our minds through the ideas we hear and the images we observe.

Once you've chosen to adopt the Mind of Christ, you must begin the daily process of protecting your newly acquired freedom. The Serpent will tirelessly barrage your Ear Gate and Eye Gate in hopes of recapturing your mind as a colony for his empire of ideas. He attacks our Ear Gates with the juiciest gossip and hypnotic lyrics, and he will even use the verbal abuse of other people for his destructive purpose.

Please be aware, your ears are sensitive and vulnerable. God uses them as a gate, too, which is another reason Scripture declares that "faith comes by hearing, and hearing by the word of God" (Romans 10:17 NKJV). But God isn't the only force making an attempt to access your mind through your Ear Gate. Everything from the conversations you entertain to the music you allow to influence your mood is vastly important.

The Serpent constantly attacks our vulnerable Eye Gates with the battering ram of negative images. Our eyes are drawn toward the Serpent's images like a driver's eye as he passes a car wreck. Thoughts of comparison begin as we observe the perfectly curated lives of other people on social media.

Our minds also get hijacked with lust and are bound by addiction as pornographic images are seen and branded onto our memories.

If all the visual content you consume on social media leaves you drained and depressed, you may want to reconsider which accounts you follow. You'll most likely need to protect your Eye Gates with unwavering accountability and develop relationships where you can be open and honest about recruiting people to help you rebuild this important gate.

Our eyes and ears have massive influence on the thoughts that occupy our mental real estate. If we seek to change our thoughts, we'll have to consider changing the stimuli of sight and sound responsible for our current mental malaise.

When the Serpent bombards our Ear Gate and Eye Gate but still can't invade the territory of our minds, a "Trojan Horse" is likely to make an appearance. It's the Serpent's last-ditch effort to undermine our ability to create a healthy mindset. It presents itself as a gift, and sometimes we're fast to reject the Serpent's knock at the doors of our ears and eyes but quick to answer as long as he masquerades in the form of a family member, loved one, romantic partner, or close friend.

Relationships can often appear as gifts. I've oftentimes lowered my defenses and opened my soul to a toxic individual. Unfortunately, by the time I realized I was dealing with a Delilah or Judas, it was too late, and a toxic soul tie had already formed. By no means would I advocate for relational isolation, but neither would I advocate for relational dysfunction. Many individuals are struggling with toxic thought patterns because of the intimate relationships that exist behind the walls of their soul. It's impossible to change your mind if you don't break soul ties with the toxic people in your life.

I have personally dealt with a plethora of "Trojan Horses," and breaking those soul ties may possibly be the most difficult task found within the pages of this book. After being married for two years, I realized my mother's toxicity was affecting the way I thought about my wife. She and I had always been close because we needed each other to overcome the challenges associated with my father's addiction. But I didn't realize that our bond would need to break in order for me to form a new bond with Tia.

The Bible is clear that "a man leaves his father and mother and is united to his wife, and they become one flesh" (Genesis 2:24). My mother wasn't necessarily the biggest fan of the woman I chose to spend the rest of my life with, and moreover, she became vocal about that. During those first two years of marriage, I would call her and then inevitably begin to feel the gravitational pull of the relationship. Then soon after, I'd be orbiting my mother's negative opinions regarding my wife. Then for the next week I would be secretly battling against negative thoughts related to Tia and our marriage because I had a toxic soul tie that needed to be broken.

So I made a painful, difficult, and mature decision. I created boundaries with my mother, and if she didn't abide by the rules of those boundaries, I simply would not speak to her. Toxic soul ties can't be managed; they must be ruthlessly broken. I came to the realization that I had never entered into a binding covenant with my mother, but I had stood before God and entered into a binding covenant with my wife. God would judge me as a husband far more harshly than He would ever judge me as a son.

The decision to break soul ties with my mother has caused both of us pain, but I no longer struggle with thoughts of doubt, fear, or regret when it comes to my marriage, and the peace of mind and mental clarity are proof that I made the correct decision.

Many of us battle with anxiety, and the source is truly internal. Others, however, are triggered toward anxiety because of the relationships in their lives. Some of us are in the storm of anxiety because Jonah is on our boat, and the only way to survive is to throw him overboard (Jonah 1:1–13). That may sound cruel, but God couldn't send a great fish to save Jonah until those sailors threw him overboard. Whenever you remove someone from your life, you're actually giving God an opportunity to sweep in and rescue them. I had to realize that God is the only one who should have a Messiah complex, and that He loves my mother more than I ever could. If anyone was going to rescue her, it would be Jesus, not me.

My prayer is that you will defend your mind against every "Trojan Horse" and put extra reinforcements at your Ear Gate and Eye Gate.

Offensive Playbook

Throughout the course of this book, we've made the long and arduous trek from the Mind of Adam to the Mind of Christ. We've regained territory that was previously inhabited by fear, anxiety, and insecurity. We've reclaimed mental property and evicted mindsets that have been squatting in our sacred spaces. The fight isn't over, though. Now that we've gained mental freedom and claimed mental clarity, we must defend it.

In a fascinating passage of Scripture, Jesus talks about the aftermath of evicting negativity from our lives and how the freedom can be short-lived if we aren't careful.

> When an impure spirit comes out of a person, it goes through arid places seeking rest and does not find it. Then it says, "I will return to the house I left." When it arrives, it finds the house unoccupied, swept clean and put in order. Then it goes and takes with it seven other spirits more wicked than itself, and they go in and live there. And the final condition of that person is worse than the first. (Matthew 12:43–45)

Along this journey we've gentrified entire neighborhoods of mental real estate, and the displaced occupants aren't happy. In Matthew 12, Jesus taught His disciples that gaining freedom is a lot easier than keeping freedom. Every demonic, toxic, and displaced mindset is eagerly looking for an opportunity to regain a foothold in the neighborhood of your mind. Jesus teaches that the spirits of doubt, fear, anxiety, and depression will eventually miss the comfortable hosting home that many of us used to provide, and those spirits will return to reclaim our minds as their space.

At first glance, this passage of Scripture may seem confusing or even disappointing because it sounds like Jesus is declaring that we're doomed and there's nothing we can do to prevent "the final condition" being "worse than the first." But Jesus isn't saying this outcome is inevitable. He teaches us how to prevent the evicted squatters from returning with a vengeance and taking over our minds again.

One key word—*unoccupied*—unlocks this entire passage of teaching. Jesus says that everything we've evicted will indeed return, and if those previous dwelling places are found to be unoccupied, then the space will inevitably be reclaimed. Which means that joy, peace, and wisdom must now reside in the homes where the Serpent had established strongholds of fear, doubt, and insecurity. The goal of this book isn't simply to help you evict toxic thoughts but to help you find and fill your mind with the tenants of peace, identity, joy, and confidence. The unoccupied mind will never stay unoccupied, but you get to decide what you will think about, and like in basketball, the best defense is a killer offense.

The unfortunate truth is that many people read the Bible as an endless list of "do nots" and sins to avoid. While commandments for our protection are certainly in there, God knows humans don't play defense nearly as well as we play offense. So most of His Word is filled with action items to accomplish instead of sins to avoid. Simply put, there are more "do" statements than "do not" statements, and Paul certainly takes this approach when telling the Philippian church how to regain control over their thoughts.

He wisely declares, "Whatever is true, whatever is noble, whatever is right, whatever is pure, whatever is lovely, whatever is admirable, if anything is excellent or praiseworthy—think about such things" (Philippians 4:8). We must be actively using our minds for the glory of God. Paul's command is to fill our minds with so many true, pure, lovely, admirable, excellent, and praiseworthy thoughts that toxic thoughts have no space to squat or footholds to win.

My parents have told me that, when I was a young kid, I was incredibly hyperactive with a seemingly endless supply of energy. They would pick me up from school and bring me straight home, and then I would either get into trouble or have issues falling asleep. For months they didn't know how to deal with their restless and mischievous young son.

Then one afternoon after my dad picked me up from school, he decided to stop at the local park before taking me home. For nearly two hours he allowed me to run around, have fun, enjoy life, and burn off all that excess energy. Once we got home, I was obedient and ready for our nightly routine. There was no mischievous activity and no restless tension because my dad had given me an outlet for all that energy.

We start every single day with a remarkable amount of mental energy that should be going toward solving the world's greatest and most complex problems, dreaming possibilities, imagining how the kingdom of God should look on Earth, creating futures, and thinking through God's divine strategy for our personal dilemmas. By evening, our minds should be so tired from dreaming, creating, and problem-solving that no energy should be left for insecurities to speak. I wonder how many of us entertain negative thoughts because we're mentally bored and underworked.

Paul also says to "set your minds on things above" in a very active and intentional way. Instead of having a passive relationship with our minds, we're supposed to put our minds to work every day as a tool to be used and a resource to be depleted. The Bible provides clear, practical, and wise counsel. If we are to maintain our mental freedom, we must occupy our minds with substantive thoughts that bring life. We are to fill them with thoughts of God and Scripture, and we're to intentionally set our minds in the direction of our destiny.

Paul avoided using the word *not* when giving advice on how to operate the Mind of Christ. He knew the best way to not think about insecurities was to fill our minds with the truth of our identities. The best way to avoid thoughts of doubt is to let faith and wonder occupy our minds. And the best way to stop thinking about our problems is to set our minds on the solution.

Don't get stuck playing defense for so long that you forget to score. Defense is important but not to the detriment of our offense. Defend your gates and occupy your mind.

If You Give a Roommate Some Toothpaste

Thanks to my parents' Sam's Club membership, I had piles of toiletries going into my freshman year of college. My dorm room was fully stocked and prepared for everything from final exams to a minor famine. I had more than enough laundry detergent, toothpaste, and ramen noodles, so I didn't make a fuss when I noticed that my roommate was helping himself to my supply of toothpaste. I didn't want to seem like a selfishly spoiled only child, so I just let it slide and reassured myself that God would reward me for my generosity.

A couple of weeks into school, though, my roommate had some sort of technical difficulty with his laptop. Honestly, I didn't listen to all the details because I didn't foresee his problem becoming my problem. So I was caught completely off guard when I entered our room one afternoon to find him on my side, at my desk, using my laptop for his homework assignments. I mustered up every ounce of politeness within my soul and simply said, "No worries, man" as he explained that he needed my laptop for the next hour. Every passive-aggressive tendency within me wanted to change the password to my laptop that night, but I didn't. I was conflicted. I wanted to be a good friend, plus my roommate was really popular, so I compromised healthy boundaries in the name of generosity.

I was in the middle of enjoying Gordon College's famous chicken fingers when I saw my roommate walk into the cafeteria. It was completely normal to bump into each other there as we crisscrossed campus on our way to classes. But when he got closer, something appeared different. I just couldn't tell what was "off" about his appearance until he got really close and approached me for a greeting.

He was wearing my pants.

I lost it. All the anger and frustration I'd been suppressing erupted to the surface, and I looked and sounded insane as I demanded that he take off my pants immediately. That seemed completely logical at the time. In hindsight, though, I'm glad he refused to strip down to his undergarments in our cafeteria. My privacy and boundaries had been violated, but I was the only one to blame for that.

The Serpent never shows up wearing your pants. Rather, he starts with small areas that seem insignificant, and the cycle of compromise begins. He can't be appeased or pacified, and he doesn't respect truces or mutually beneficial agreements. If the Serpent is given a foothold in your mind, it won't be long until the two of you are inhabiting the same space.

If you've ever read *If You Give a Mouse a Cookie* by Laura Numeroff, you've seen the power of the Serpent's slippery slope of compromise beautifully illustrated. Once the mouse gets a cookie, he wants more. The Serpent will never be satisfied with a foothold, toothpaste, or a cookie, and if you give him one thought, it will always lead to another.

But if the Mind of Christ has taught us anything, it's to be vigilant over every square inch of mental real estate we have and to fill it daily with God-thoughts and heavenly ideas.

In Conclusion

If you've taken the journey to the Mind of Christ, allowing our Lord to wash your brain, I pray it has changed you as much as the destination will bless you. I pray that you'll use every tool we've discussed. I pray that the glory of God will be revealed through the instrument of your mind. I pray that you will go forth in courage and curiosity to help create the colony of heaven here on Earth. I pray that you will begin to think about *what* you think about and that your thoughts will serve you well as you accomplish God's plan for your life.

And lastly, I pray you'll become a guide for someone else who's still stuck in mental bondage.

Acknowledgments

PASTOR ANDY THOMPSON, I could never repay you for how you've invested in my life. You taught me how to be a man. Love you, Pop.

Andrew Damazio, the day you showed me your father's books in your office changed my life. No exaggeration. My prayer is that my son, Theo, will one day show my books to his friends. Love you, man.

To Pastors Robert and Taylor Madu, thanks for opening your world and your church to the Arango family. Pastor Robert, you've been a friend, brother, mentor, coach, and more. Love you.

To my agent, Tom Dean, you are an answer to prayer. Thanks for seeing my potential as an author. I appreciate you more than I could express.

To my line editor, Jean Kavich Bloom, you took my words and my voice and removed all the blemishes. I could never thank you enough.

Stephanie Smith, you are a woman of your word. The moment you prayed over this project during our Zoom meeting was a game changer. Thanks so much.

To the entire Manny Arango Ministries team—Deborah, Elijah, Jayon, Jordan, Sam, Daniel, Will, and Tia. We're changing the world. One sermon at a time. One course at a time. One book at a time. Thanks for believing in me. Thanks for trusting me. Thanks for entertaining all my crazy ideas.

Notes

Chapter 1 Doubt Takes the Lead

1. A.W. Tozer, *The Knowledge of the Holy* (San Francisco: HarperOne, 1978), 1.
2. Dallas Willard, *Renovation of the Heart* (Colorado Springs, CO: The Navigators, 2014), 100.
3. Willard, *Renovation of the Heart*, 100.
4. Tozer, *The Knowledge of the Holy*, 1.

Chapter 4 Just Talking?

1. "dictator," https://www.etymonline.com/word/dictator.

Chapter 5 The Maker's Mark

1. Sam Johnson, "How Much Did Famous Logos Cost to Design," FreeYork, https://freeyork.org/art/much-famous-logos-cost/.
2. Alix Spiegel, "Teachers' Expectations Can Influence How Students Perform," *Morning Edition*, September 17, 2012, https://www.npr.org/sections/health-shots/2012/09/18/161159263/teachers-expectations-can-influence-how-students-perform.
3. "metanoia," https://www.merriam-webster.com/dictionary/metanoia.

Chapter 6 Designed for Connection

1. Johann Hari, "Everything You Think You Know About Addiction Is Wrong," TED: Ideas Worth Sharing, May 2014, https://www.ted.com/talks/johann_hari_everything_you_think_you_know_about_addiction_is_wrong.
2. Bruce K. Alexander, "Addiction: The View from Rat Pack" (2010), https://brucekalexander.com/articles-speeches/rat-park/148-addiction-the-view-from-rat-park.
3. "The Portugal Drug Policy," bePortugal, https://beportugal.com/portugal-drug-laws/.

Chapter 8 Don't Feed the Monkeys

1. Timothy Keller with Kathy Keller, *The Meaning of Marriage* (New York, NY: Penguin Publishing Group, 2013), 101.
2. Keller, *The Meaning of Marriage*, 101.

About the Author

Manny Arango is a preacher, a Bible nerd, a storyteller, and an overcomer. He's passionate about fighting for people who have lost their voice and lost their way.

Manny is a teaching pastor at Social Dallas, and also speaks at conferences and other gatherings across the globe. He deeply values biblical literacy and recently founded ARMA (Latin for "armor"), a ministry that offers original online courses about the Bible and theology.

Manny previously served as a teaching pastor at World Overcomers Christian Church, a multicultural megachurch in Durham, North Carolina, and before that he served as the youth pastor at World Overcomers.

He graduated from Southeastern University with his master's degree and is currently in a doctoral program at Northern Seminary. Manny has been married to his loving wife, Tia, since 2014. After several years of struggling with infertility, they welcomed a son in 2021.